OTHER BOOKS BY DR. MARGARET R. O'LEARY AND DR. DENNIS S. O'LEARY

Tragedy at Graignes: The Bud Sophian Story (2011)

Adventures at Wohelo Camp: Summer of 1928 (2011)

R. D. O'Leary: Notes from Oxford, 1910–1911 (2014)

R. D. O'Leary: Notes from Mount Oread, 1914–1915 (2015)

Raphael Dorman O'Leary: The English Professor (2016)

The Texas Meningitis Epidemic 1911–1913: Origin of the Meningococcal Vaccine (2018)

THE KANSAS CITY MENINGITIS EPIDEMIC, 1911–1913:

Violent and Not Imagined

Margaret R. O'Leary, MD

Dennis S. O'Leary, MD

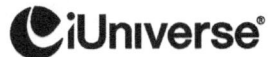

THE KANSAS CITY MENINGITIS EPIDEMIC, 1911-1913:
VIOLENT AND NOT IMAGINED

iUniverse books may be ordered through booksellers or by contacting:

iUniverse
1663 Liberty Drive
Bloomington, IN 47403
www.iuniverse.com
1-800-Authors (1-800-288-4677)

Because of the dynamic nature of the Internet, any web addresses or
links contained in this book may have changed since publication and
may no longer be valid. The views expressed in this work are solely those
of the author and do not necessarily reflect the views of the publisher,
and the publisher hereby disclaims any responsibility for them.

Any people depicted in stock imagery provided by Getty Images are
models, and such images are being used for illustrative purposes only.
Certain stock imagery © Getty Images.

ISBN: 978-1-5320-6231-5 (sc)
ISBN: 978-1-5320-6232-2 (hc)
ISBN: 978-1-5320-6230-8 (e)

Library of Congress Control Number: 2018913296

Print information available on the last page.

iUniverse rev. date: 02/15/2019

CONTENTS

PREFACE

The Kansas City Meningitis Epidemic, 1911–1913: Violent and Not Imagined is the historical account of one city's harrowing struggle against an epidemic of cerebrospinal meningitis. Before the 1940s, when antibiotics first became available to cure this disease, a cerebrospinal meningitis epidemic was one of the most malignant, rapacious, nondiscriminating, unpredictable, and difficult-to-control contagious-disease epidemics afflicting humans. The epidemic in Kansas City described in this book was no exception.

The Kansas City cerebrospinal meningitis epidemic piqued our interest because of the contributions to its control by Dr. Abraham Sophian, a celebrated American public health clinician and researcher. He also was a commanding, distinguished, fastidious, and tireless internist in Kansas City during the first half of the twentieth century, as well as the maternal grandfather of one of us (Dr. Dennis Sophian O'Leary). We first learned about his involvement in the Kansas City cerebrospinal meningitis epidemic during our research into the even more ferocious, contemporaneous Texas cerebrospinal meningitis epidemic of 1911 to 1913, as described elsewhere.[1]

We have devoted many years of our lives to the direct and indirect care of patients suffering from severe diseases, such as cerebrospinal meningitis—one of us in emergency medicine (Dr. Margaret Rose O'Leary) and the other in internal medicine (Dr. Dennis S. O'Leary). We have written copiously—both separately and together—for all of our professional lives as physicians. During our almost forty years of marriage, writing has been a shared rewarding experience for us.

Telling the story of the Kansas City cerebrospinal meningitis epidemic of 1911 to 1913 involves technical concepts and terminology that might be new to some readers. We have introduced the book with a brief history of knowledge of cerebrospinal meningitis to facilitate readers' understanding of the events of the Kansas City cerebrospinal meningitis epidemic of 1911 to 1913. Carefully reading the introduction will probably be a good investment for most readers.

Of note, this book describes the cerebrospinal meningitis epidemic in Kansas City, Missouri, and not the contemporaneous epidemic in the contiguous city of Kansas City, Kansas. The latter city, which equally suffered and responded heroically, deserves separate treatment. Of the two cities, Kansas City, Missouri, was (and is) by far the much larger, with a population in 1910 of about 250,000 people.[2] The population of Kansas City, Kansas, in the same year was around 82,000 people.[3] Whenever we use the name Kansas City in this book, we are referring to Kansas City, Missouri, unless otherwise noted.

For the purpose of this book, the adjectives "communicable," "infectious," "contagious," and "transmissible," as used to modify the word disease, mean the same thing—that is, a specific disease, such as cerebrospinal meningitis, is capable of traveling from one person to another. Different jurisdictions in the United States during the past century have used one or another of these adjectives to describe their experiences.

Margaret R. O'Leary, MD
Dennis S. O'Leary, MD
Fairway, Kansas
October 12, 2018

PREFACE NOTES

1. Margaret R. O'Leary and Dennis S. O'Leary, *The Texas Meningitis Epidemic, 1911–1913: Origin of the Meningococcal Vaccine* (Bloomington, IN: iUniverse, 2018).
2. United States Bureau of the Census, "Table 14, Population of the 100 Largest Urban Places: 1910," accessed May 22, 2018, https://www.census.gov/population/www/documentation/twps0027/tab14.txt.
3. "Population of Cities in Kansas, 1900–2010," KU Institute for Policy and Social Research, University of Kansas, accessed May 31, 2018, http://www.ipsr.ku.edu/ksdata/ksah/population/2pop33.pdf.

ACKNOWLEDGMENTS

We appreciate the assistance of the following people in the preparation of this book: Sister Mary Kay Liston, CSJ, D. Min., archivist, Truman Medical Center-Hospital Hill, Kansas City, Missouri; Elizabeth Shepard, interim head of archives, Archives of New York-Presbyterian/Weill Cornell, New York City, New York; Rebecca Schulte, associate librarian and university archivist, Kenneth Spencer Research Library, University of Kansas Libraries, Lawrence, Kansas; Kathy A. Lafferty, copy services manager and reference, Kenneth Spencer Research Library, University of Kansas Libraries, Lawrence, Kansas; Michael Wells, Missouri Valley Special Collections Librarian, Kansas City Public Library, Kansas City, Missouri; Mitch Sumner, Missouri University Libraries, University of Missouri, Kansas City, Missouri; the library staff at the LaBudde Special Collections Library, Miller Nichols Library, University of Missouri, Kansas City; the library staff at the Missouri Valley Special Collections, Kansas City Public Library, Kansas City, Missouri; Dawn McInnis, rare book librarian, Clendening History of Medicine Library, University of Kansas Medical Center, Kansas City, Kansas; Teri Watkins, senior publishing services associate, iUniverse, Bloomington, Indiana; and Alison Holen, artist and cover design supervisor, WestBow Press.

A BRIEF HISTORY OF CEREBROSPINAL MENINGITIS AND ITS TREATMENT, 1805-1908

Between October 1911 and June 1913, a brutal epidemic of cerebrospinal meningitis swept through Texas and up into Oklahoma, Missouri, and Kansas, killing thousands of people in its wake. This epidemic occurred about a century after Dr. Gaspard Vieusseux[1] provided the first known description of a cerebrospinal meningitis epidemic, which occurred in Geneva, Switzerland, in February, March, and April of 1805.[2-3] The distinctive and lethal nature of the disease startled the region's physicians. One of them, Dr. Vieusseux, wrote,

> Though the illness that reigned during the recent spring in and around Geneva was not considerable by the number of those afflicted and those who died [there were thirty-three deaths] and that endured for three months before disappearing in the summer, it nevertheless was remarkable by the symptoms that distinguished it from all the other fevers that

presented to physicians who had exercised their art in their cities for more than 30 years.[2]

Dr. Vieusseux continued,

> The outbreak began in a suspicious and scary manner a very small distance from the city in a disease in a dirty quarter habituated by poor people and others vulnerable to the development of all contagious diseases ... At the end of January [1805], in a family composed of a woman and three children, two of the children were attacked and died in less than 48 hours.

Dr. Vieusseux described the disease's clinical presentation:

> There appears suddenly a severe prostration, accompanied by a feeble pulse—small and fast, sometimes almost gone, and in a few cases, hard and elevated. It manifests itself with a violent headache, especially over the forehead, followed by heart pain or the vomiting of greenish material [and] of stiffness of the spine. In the fatal cases, the course was extremely rapid, lasting only 12 hours in some cases, in others from one to five days. In children there were convulsions. In those who died within 24 hours of the onset, the larger proportion had an eruption of violet spots[4] upon the body.[2]

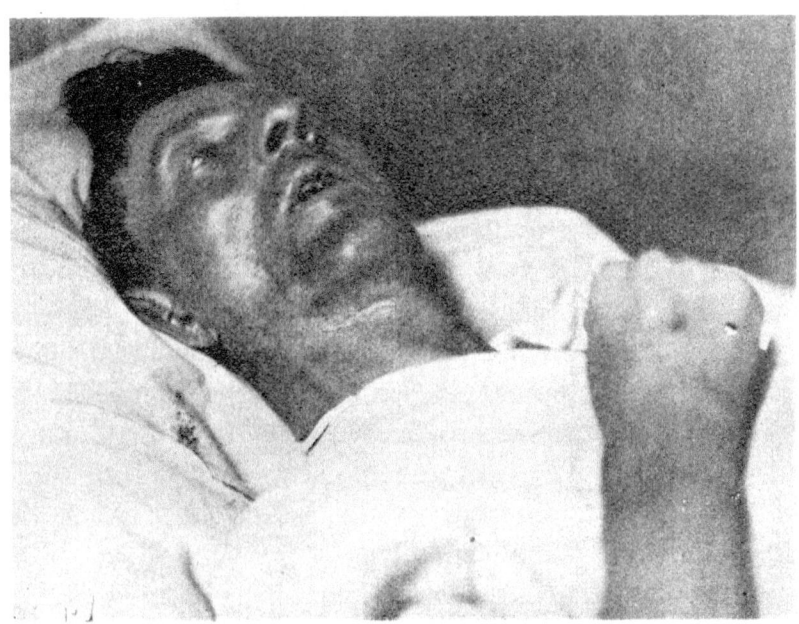

A male patient with cerebrospinal meningitis. The original caption accompanying this image is: "An alcoholic patient, ill thirty-six hours with epidemic meningitis. Violently delirious and deeply stuporous at intervals. Note the blank expression and the rigidity of the neck." The photographer is unknown. The image and caption are from Abraham Sophian, *Epidemic Cerebrospinal Meningitis* (St. Louis, MO: C. V. Mosby, 1913), 74.

The disease quickly crossed the Atlantic Ocean to infect communities in the eastern United States. Dr. Elisha North[5] described an epidemic in Goshen, Litchfield County, Connecticut, in 1806, as "a flood of mighty waters, bringing along the horrors of a most dreadful plague."[6-7] The same year, Dr. Lothario Danielson[8] and Dr. Elias Mann[9] described a similar "singular and very mortal disease" epidemic in Medfield, Norfolk County, Massachusetts, during which nine people died between March 8, 1806, and March 31, 1806. The two physicians noted, "The patient is suddenly taken with violent pain in the head and stomach succeeded by cold chills and followed by nausea and puking." The autopsies of five victims revealed adherent meninges (coverings of the brain and spinal cord) exuding pus.[10]

In 1847, Dr. François Louis Isidore Valleix[11] in Paris termed the disease "simple acute meningitis" to distinguish it from "tuberculosis of the meninges."[12] Simple acute meningitis lacked antecedent symptoms; launched violently with a severe headache, photophobia, and frequent vomiting; and progressed rapidly and continuously over one to six days (rarely longer) before terminating in death, without perceptible remissions. Tuberculosis of the meninges had clear antecedent symptoms of tubercular disease, such as cough, fever, night sweats, and weight loss (i.e., symptoms associated with pulmonary tuberculosis); presented insidiously with mild symptoms; and progressed slowly and discontinuously (with remissions) for weeks and months before terminating in death.[12] In 1872, no one knew the cause of either simple acute meningitis or tubercular meningitis.

Two decades passed, as cerebrospinal meningitis continued its deadly forays into cities and towns in the United States, frustrating physicians who were helpless to alleviate the intense suffering of their afflicted patients. In 1868, Dr. Meredith Clymer,[13] the estimable physician of Philadelphia and New York City, renamed simple acute meningitis as "cerebrospinal meningitis," describing it as

> an acute specific disorder, commonly happening as an epidemic, general or limited, and, rarely, sporadically; caused by some unknown external influence; of sudden onset, rapid course, and very fatal; its chief symptoms, referable to the cerebrospinal axis are great prostration of the vital powers, severe pain in the head and along the spinal column, delirium, tetanic, and occasionally clonic, spasms, and cutaneous hyperaesthesia, with, in some cases, stupor, coma, and motor paralysis; attended frequently with cutaneous haemic spots; its morbid anatomical characters being congestion and inflammation of the membranes of the brain and spinal cord, particularly the pia mater, although there is reason to believe that the evidence of these

4

changes may be wanting, even in cases of long duration.[14]

In 1872, a fierce cerebrospinal meningitis epidemic struck the old city of New York City (the present boroughs of Manhattan and the Bronx), killing 782 residents. (Henceforth, New York City refers to the Manhattan and Bronx boroughs combined unless otherwise noted). Epidemiologically-speaking, the number 782 is called a *death count*. Health officials obtained the death count number in every way possible, including by death certificates, by report of physicians and institutions, and by complaints of citizens and others.

Cerebrospinal meningitis was not a reportable disease in 1872, so New York City health department officials lacked information about the total number of persons with the disease (the total number of persons with the disease includes both those people who had died from the disease and those who had survived it). However, health department officials did know that the population size of New York City in 1872 was 968,710 residents.[14] With this information, they divided the death count (782) by the size of the population (968,710) to produce a mortality rate of *8.07 meningitis deaths per 10,000 New York City residents*.[15] The mortality rate allowed health department officials to compare the disease's death impact across populations, places, times, and other diseases.

Meanwhile, the cause of cerebrospinal meningitis during the epidemic of 1872 in New York City remained elusive. Dr. Clymer, expressing the consensus of his peers, noted that disease's cause was "beyond physical and bodily conditions [and was] outside of the degree of heat, moisture, etc., and the constitutional state of the individual." He concluded, "We are forced to take refuge in the assumption of an unknown special morbific agent as the aetic factor."[16]

Another decade passed. In 1882, bacteriologist Dr. Robert Koch[17] in Berlin first identified the tubercle bacillus (*Mycobacterium tuberculosis*), an acid-fast[18] microorganism, as the cause of tuberculosis. His discovery finally settled the question of the cause of tubercular meningitis. Three years later (1885), bacteriologist

Dr. Anton Weichselbaum[19] at the University of Vienna, identified a Gram-negative[20] microorganism as the cause of cerebrospinal meningitis. He named the microorganism *Diplococcus intracellularis meningitidis* after its tendency to reside in flattened pairs inside the inflammatory cells of infected cerebrospinal fluid. Dr. Weichselbaum isolated the meningococcus from six of the eight specimens of cerebrospinal fluid submitted to him by Central European physicians who had collected them from their patients with meningitis.[21] Dr. Weichselbaum published his discovery in *Fortschritte der Medizin* in 1887.[22] In 1901, Dr. Heinrich Albrecht and Dr. Anton Ghon renamed Weichselbaum's microorganism *Neisseria meningitides*, the moniker that holds today.[23]

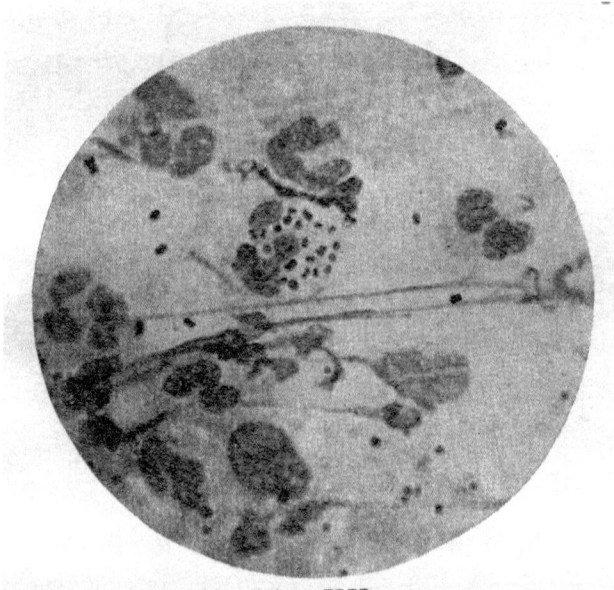

Fig. XX.

Meningococci and inflammatory cells in a drop of cerebrospinal fluid as seen through a microscopic lens, 1912–1913. The original caption of this image was: "Stained sediment of cerebrospinal fluid removed from a case of epidemic meningitis at the beginning of the disease, before serum treatment was instituted. Note the presence of intra- and extracellular diplococci and pus-cells." The image was scanned from Abraham Sophian, *Epidemic Cerebrospinal Meningitis* (St. Louis, MO: C. V. Mosby, 1913), 245. The photographer is unknown.

Nearly two more decades passed after the discovery of the *Neisseria meningitidis* bacterium, also known as the meningococcus. In 1904, New York City suffered its worst cerebrospinal meningitis epidemic in terms of loss of life since the cerebrospinal meningitis epidemic of 1872.[24] Of the 2,318,831 New York City residents in 1904, 1,083 succumbed to the disease, resulting in a mortality rate of *4.6 meningitis deaths per 10,000 New York City residents.*[24] The mortality rates for cerebrospinal meningitis in New York City for the years 1866 through 1907 are listed in the following table. The bolded numbers are mentioned in the text.

Table 1: Number of Cases and Deaths from, Cerebrospinal Meningitis in the Old City of New York (Present Boroughs Manhattan and Bronx), 1866–1907, Inclusive[24]

Year	Population (Manhattan and the Bronx combined)	No. of Deaths from Cerebrospinal Meningitis	Mortality Rate per 10,000
1866	767,979	18	.23
1867	808,489	33	.40
1868	851,137	34	.39
1869	896,034	42	.47
1870	943,300	32	.34
1871	955,921	48	.50
1872	**968,710**	**782**	**8.07**
1873	981,671	290	2.95
1874	1,030,607	158	1.53
1875	1,044,396	146	1.40
1876	1,075,532	127	1.18
1877	1,107,597	116	1.05
1878	1,140,617	97	.85
1879	1,174,621	108	.92

1880	1,209,196	170	1.41
1881	1,244,511	461	3.70
1882	1,288,857	238	1.86
1883	1,390,388	223	1.69
1884	1,356,764	210	1.55
1885	1,396,388	202	1.45
1886	1,437,170	223	1.55
1887	1,479,143	203	1.37
1888	1,522,341	173	1.14
1889	1,566,801	145	.93
1890	1,612,559	136	.84
1891	1,659,654	189	1.14
1892	1,708,124	230	1.35
1893	1,758,010	469	2.67
1894	1,809,353	213	1.18
1895	1,873,201	204	1.09
1896	1,906,139	178	.93
1897	1,940,553	232	1.20
1898	1,976,572	258	1.31
1899	2,014,330	287	1.42
1900	2,055,714	201	.97
1901	2,118,209	201	.94
1902	2,182,836	190	.87
1903	2,249,680	195	.86
1904	2,318,831	1,083	4.60
1905	2,390,382	1,511	6.30
1906	2,464,432	600	2.50
1907	2,541,471	471	1.80

In 1904, physicians still did not know how cerebrospinal meningitis was transmitted. However, in general, they believed that it was not highly contagious. For example, Bellevue Hospital[25] physicians in 1904 year admitted persons afflicted with cerebrospinal meningitis to the hospital's general wards, reasoning that the disease was only mildly contagious and that no afflicted patient had ever communicated his or her disease to a Bellevue physician or nurse, with one exception. That exception was Dr. Joseph F. McCarthy,[26] an attending physician and Bellevue Hospital who contracted the disease and became a patient at Bellevue Hospital but did not know how he had acquired the disease.[27] Dr. Thomas Darlington,[28] the New York City health commissioner in 1904, concurred with the Bellevue physicians' assessment, proclaiming that cerebrospinal meningitis was not "directly contagious," and "if meningitis [was] contagious it [was] in slight degree."[29]

The next year (1905), cerebrospinal meningitis returned with a vengeance to New York City, killing 1,511 persons of the 2,390,382 persons making up the population that year. The mortality rate calculated to *6.3 deaths per 10,000 New York City residents*, as compared with the mortality rate of *4.60 per 10,000 New York City residents* the previous year (1904) (see Table 1).[24] The disease also erupted in other cities in 1905, including Philadelphia, where it killed Dr. Albert Burns Craig.[30] The death of this relatively young Philadelphia physician and the rising death count and mortality rate associated with cerebrospinal meningitis in New York City between 1904 and 1905 so alarmed Dr. Darlington that he convened a New York City commission[31] of medical experts[32] to study the disease. The medical experts included Dr. Simon Flexner,[33] director of the fledgling Rockefeller Institute for Medical Research,[34] and Dr. Hermann Michael Biggs,[35] the chief medical officer of the New York City Board of Health[36] and its Research Laboratory.[37] Dr. Darlington tasked the commission with evaluating the disease's degree of communicability, its modes of transmission, and the possibilities for its control.

Dr. Flexner determined, through experimentation with his laboratory monkeys, that cerebrospinal meningitis was indeed contagious.[38] Dr. Charles Bolduan,[39] a bacteriologist with the Research Laboratory, confirmed earlier studies that identified a healthy meningococcal carrier state. This state was identified through the culturing of meningococci from the noses and throats of healthy individuals during cerebrospinal meningitis epidemics.[40] A theory of infection was that the meningococci entered the body by way of the nose and throat, where they lived without producing an illness, and then, in a small proportion of cases, gained access to the bloodstream, which delivered them to the meninges, where they caused meningitis.[24]

Based on the commission's findings, the New York City Board of Health declared cerebrospinal meningitis a communicable disease and henceforth "required reporting of all cases by physicians, enforcement of quarantine, isolation of patients, exclusion of other children in the family from school, and disinfection of premises and bedding on termination of the disease."[40] One case of cerebrospinal meningitis was defined as one person with cerebrospinal meningitis. Reports of cases of cerebrospinal meningitis began to flow to the New York City Board of Health, thereby making possible for the first time a *case count*. A case count consisted of a running tally of the number of cases counted. The case count provided health department officials with a better grasp of the activity of the disease. As noted above, the case count was made up of the people who had died from the disease and the people who were surviving, or had survived, the disease. The case count permitted the identification of disease patterns and control planning.

Health department officials subsequently figured out that a case count divided by the size of the population from which the case count arose could provide a frequency rate useful for comparing the extent of the disease's presence (prevalence) in different populations, places, and times. *Prevalence*[41] (prevalence rate) is the case count of all persons with a health condition in a given population during a specified period of time. For example, the cerebrospinal meningitis case count in Greater New York City in 1906 was 1,032, according to the *Journal of Experimental Medicine*.[42] Using this case count, the prevalence rate for cerebrospinal meningitis in 1906 in Greater New York City calculated to *4.2 cerebrospinal meningitis cases per 10,000 Greater New York City residents*.

As early as 1905, researchers in the United States and Europe (where the disease also was prevalent) sought a cure for cerebrospinal meningitis. The major research laboratories[43] were the Research Laboratory of the New York City Board of Health and the Rockefeller Institute for Medical Research,[44] both in New York City; the laboratory of Drs. Wilhelm Kolle and August von Wasserman at the Institute for Infectious Diseases in Berlin, Germany[45]; and the laboratory of Dr. Georg Jochmann at the Medizinische Klinik of Breslau, Germany.[46]

The cure developed by the four research laboratories was an antimeningitis serum produced by immunizing horses with the meningococcus. Dr. Flexner, after experimenting to find the safest and most humane way to immunize his horses, settled on the subcutaneous route. He injected his horses with live meningococci and autolysates (i.e., the disintegration products of meningococcal cultures) at seven-day intervals. He used many different strains of the meningococci to prepare the living cultures and autolysate. He gradually increased the dose of living meningococci injected into his horses over six to twelve months. He then harvested, purified, and bottled the horse serum for use in humans.[47]

In 1905, Dr. William Hallock Park,[48] the director of the Research Laboratory of the New York City Board of Health, sent vials of his laboratory's antimeningitis serum for subcutaneous injection in twenty desperately-ill cerebrospinal meningitis patients in Hartford, Hartford County, Connecticut. Dr. Park and the Hartford physicians requesting the antimeningitis serum for their patients hoped that it might benefit persons with cerebrospinal meningitis in the same way that subcutaneous administration of diphtheria antitoxin benefitted patients with diphtheria. Unfortunately, the use of the antimeningitis serum in Hartford produced uncertain results. As a result, Dr. Park withheld further antimeningitis serum from distribution.[43] Despite the disappointing results of the subcutaneous injection of antimeningitis serum in persons with cerebrospinal meningitis, Dr. Park never gave up the idea that the approach could work, referring to the "somewhat favorable" results achieved by Dr. Kolle and Dr. Wassermann in Berlin in their cerebrospinal meningitis patients administered subcutaneous antimeningitis serum.[49]

In April and May 1906, Dr. Georg Jochmann first experimented with the *intraspinal* injection of antimeningitis serum in thirty-eight infected persons at the Medizinische Klinik of Breslau. He injected ten to twenty cubic centimeters of antimeningitis serum directly into the inflamed meninges of his patients, noting a prompt beneficial response. During the course of the year (1906), he used the intraspinal antimeningitis serum in thirty more afflicted patients. He then compared the health outcomes of cerebrospinal meningitis patients treated with intraspinal antimeningitis serum to the cerebrospinal meningitis patients not so treated. Twenty-seven percent of his patients who received the intraspinal antimeningitis serum died, while 52 percent of his patients who did not receive the intraspinal antimeningitis serum died.[50] The administration of intraspinal antimeningitis serum apparently had rendered the disease less lethal.

The 27 percent and 52 percent figures noted above are called *lethality rates*, better known as *case fatality rates*.[41] The case fatality rate is the proportion of persons with a disease who die from it. It is calculated by dividing the death count by the case count during a specified period of time. It is always expressed as a percentage. The case fatality rate is not the same as the mortality rate, even though both rates contain the death count in their numerators. In a mortality rate, the denominator is the size of the population at risk; in a case fatality rate, the denominator is the case count of persons infected with the disease. With the advent of antimeningitis serum, the case fatality rate became an important measure of the efficacy of intraspinal antimeningitis serum in persons with cerebrospinal meningitis.

Dr. Flexner carefully followed news of Dr. Jochmann's experiments. In August 1906, he proclaimed the latter's intraspinal injection innovation premature, writing in the *Journal of the American Medical Association*, "I do not think that the injection into the spinal canal of man of alien sera should be undertaken until their physiologic action has been worked out in more detail in monkeys."[51] Dr. Flexner then tested and established to his satisfaction the efficacy and safety of the intraspinal antimeningitis serum route of administration in his laboratory monkeys. In 1907, he offered his antimeningitis serum to physicians for use in humans in New York City; Philadelphia; Cleveland, Castalia, and Akron, Ohio; Edinburgh, Scotland; and Belfast, Ireland.[52] Dr. Flexner collected outcome data on forty-seven patients with cerebrospinal meningitis who received his antimeningitis serum via the intraspinal route in these cities. Of the forty-seven persons, thirty-four (72.3 percent) recovered, and thirteen (27.6 percent) died.[53]

Dr. Flexner was pleased with the data but quickly foresaw the need for a larger human clinical test group. To accomplish this goal, he supplied antimeningitis serum free of charge directly to physicians throughout the United States and world. In return for the free antimeningitis serum, he required physicians to meet certain conditions and to return specified cerebrospinal meningitis outcome data to him.[54]

For example, Dr. Flexner requested proof that the patient receiving the antimeningitis serum had meningococcal meningitis and not some other form of meningitis (e.g., tubercular meningitis). The only way to establish the cause of meningitis was to perform a lumbar puncture procedure. This procedure consisted of inserting a long, hollow spinal needle (Quincke needle)[55] through the cleansed skin of a patient's lower back until the needle reached the cerebrospinal fluid space,[56] withdrawing a volume of cerebrospinal fluid, examining the fluid via microscopy to determine or exclude the presence of *Neisseria meningitidis*, and creating a culture of the fluid to validate the microscopic findings.

This brief history of cerebrospinal meningitis and its treatment brings us to the year 1908, whence our story opens in Kansas City. Established in 1838 at the confluence of the Missouri and Kansas Rivers, Kansas City played a major role in the westward expansion of the United States, as the Santa Fe and Oregon Trails passed through the area. During the 1870s, Kansas City was known as Cow Town because of its booming stock yards and meat packing plants.

Kansas City had limited experience with cerebrospinal meningitis before 1908. Specifically, during the cold winter months of 1898–1899, cerebrospinal meningitis visited the city's population of around 164,000 people,[57] killing twenty-six people in March 1899 (a March 1899 mortality rate of *1.59 meningitis deaths per 10,000 Kansas City residents*)[58] and between April 1, 1899, and April 14, 1899, seventeen people (a mortality rate for the first two weeks of April 1899 of *1.0 meningitis deaths per 10,000 Kansas City residents*).[59] Physicians practicing in the Kansas City area since the American Civil War stated they had never seen a case of cerebrospinal meningitis before the eruption in 1898–1899.[58]

Even though Dr. Anton Weichselbaum had identified the bacterial cause of cerebrospinal meningitis in 1885, as noted above, many Kansas City physicians in 1899 remained skeptical about his assertion. For example, Dr. Edwin Taylor Phillips,[60] a busy Kansas City physician of the era, declared, "There is probably a germ which causes the irritation, though it has never been isolated definitely. The germ theory has been carried to an unnecessary extent, it is now admitted, and it may be that meningitis is brought about by conditions not at all consistent with this theory."[58] The cerebrospinal meningitis event of 1899 and the memory of it faded with the earnest onset of warm weather.

INTRODUCTION NOTES

1. See Gaspard Vieusseux, "Mémoire sur la maladie qui a règne à Genève, au printemps de 1805," *Journal de Médecine, Chirurgie, Pharmacie, etc.*, tome xii (1806): 163–82; and "Gaspard Vieusseux; The Disease Which Raged in Geneva during the Spring of 1805," in Ralph Hermon Major, ed., *Classic Descriptions of Disease* (Springfield, IL: Charles C. Thomas, 1959), 188–90.

2. Dr. Gaspar Vieusseux (1746–1814), a native of Geneva, Switzerland, obtained his medical doctorate from the University of Leiden, South Holland, Netherlands, in 1766. After studying medicine in both Edinburgh and London, he returned to Geneva to practice medicine in 1770. He quickly embraced smallpox vaccination as a preventive or mitigator of the disease and published *Traité de la Nouvelle Méthode d'Inoculer La Petite Vérole* in 1773. He was practicing smallpox vaccination twenty-three years before Dr. Edward Jenner (1749–1823) "discovered" the practice in England. In 1805, twenty-seven-year-old Dr. Vieusseux gave the first modern description of what is now known as cerebrospinal meningitis in "Mémoire sur la maladie qui a règne à Genève, au printemps de 1805," which he published in the *Journal de Médecine, Chirurgie, Pharmacie, etc.*, tome xii (1806): 163–82, as noted above. On January 4, 1808, at the age of sixty-two years, he developed a neurological syndrome consisting of vertigo, unilateral facial numbness, loss of pain and temperature appreciation in the opposite limbs, dysphasia and hoarseness, minor tongue involvement, hiccups, and drop of an eyelid. He visited London in 1810–1811 and communicated his clinical situation to his friend Dr. Alexander Marcet (1770–1822), a native of Geneva who lived in London. Dr. Marcet published Dr. Vieusseux's communication in "History of a Singular Nervous or Paralytic Affection, Attended with Anomalous Morbid Sensations, Communicated by Dr. Marcet, Read Dec. 18, 1810," *Medico-Chirurgical Transactions* 2 (1811): 215–33. Dr. Vieusseux had another stroke in 1813 and died in the fall of 1814 at the age of forty-eight years.

3. A history of meningitis in Geneva, Switzerland, prior to Dr. Vieusseux's description in 1806 is available in Eduard-Rudolf Müllener, "Six Geneva Physicians on Meningitis," *Journal of the History of Medicine and Allied Sciences* 20, no. 1 (January 1965): 1–26. See also R. Bruce Low, "Epidemic Cerebrospinal Meningitis,"

Transactions of the Epidemiological Society of London, New Series 18 (January 20, 1899): 53–85.

4. Physicians as early as Dr. Vieusseux in 1806 noted that some patients in whom they otherwise suspected cerebrospinal meningitis because of fever and headache developed a violet-colored pinprick (petechial) rash that spread over most of their bodies. This set of patients usually died within twenty-four to forty-eight hours. In the early 1940s, physicians called this disease entity meningococcemia, meaning a blood infection with *Neisseria meningitidis*. Some researchers now attribute the rash of meningococcemia to a heavy bacterial load of meningococci entering the bloodstream, spreading and colonizing peripheral blood vessels, and leaking out of the vasculature into the surrounding tissues. The leakage produces the petechiae (one- or two-millimeter red or purple skin spots), which might also coalesce to form purpura, or pools of blood beneath the skin. On account of this petechial rash, cerebrospinal meningitis has been called spotted fever, petechial fever, purpuric fever, neuro-purpuric fever, purpura maligna, infectious purpura, purpura contagiosis, purple fever, and malignant purple fever. See Mathieu Coureuil, Olivier Join-Lambert, Hervé Lécuyer, et al., "Pathogenesis of Meningococcemia," *Cold Spring Harbor Perspectives in Medicine* 3, no. 6 (June 2013): a012393.

5. Dr. Elisha North (1771–1843) was born in Goshen, Litchfield County, Connecticut, about fifty miles west of Hartford, as one of the nine children of Dr. Joseph North Jr. (1737–1806) and Lucy Cole (1747–1829). He studied medicine with his father and Dr. Lemuel Hopkins of Hartford. He then practiced medicine in Goshen to earn money to attend the University of Pennsylvania School of Medicine in 1793, where he studied under Dr. Benjamin Rush (1746–1813). He returned to Goshen before earning his medical diploma and resumed his medical practice. Epidemic cerebrospinal meningitis was a new and obscure disease when it struck Goshen during the winters of 1806–1807 and 1808–1809. Dr. North wrote about the epidemic in *A Treatise on a Malignant Epidemic Commonly Called Spotted Fever* (New York: T. and J. Swords, 1811), an early American medical classic. He described the clinical findings of the disease as follows: "A great, surprising, and sudden loss of strength, is a constant and prominent symptom ... Violent pain of the head, and many times of the limbs, is among the first symptoms ... There is loss of appetite, and sickness at stomach, and vomiting." He added, "The worst

form this disease ever assumes, particularly in children, is that of coma, or cholera morbus. It frequently assumes the form of a violent mania at the time, or within a few hours of the attack, particularly in sanguine young men. Sometimes delirium is among the first symptoms; sometimes coma; and many times, petechiae." Dr. North described petechiae as variable in size and in color, from a bright red to a bright purple. He did not believe the presence of petechiae occurred often enough to warrant naming the disease after them. He said, "Unless the patient recovers, he commonly dies within the first 12, 24, or 48 hours. Death is ushered in by the gradual giving up of the powers of life, by syncope, by the febrile apoplexy, or by convulsions." He noted that the appearance of petechiae marked the worst form of the disease and that petechiae occurred in almost every case during the 1806–1807 Goshen epidemic but only rarely in the 1808–1809 Goshen epidemic. Dr. North married Hannah Beach (1775–1862); they had eight children. He died at the age of seventy-two years. See "Elisha North," in Ralph Hermon Major, ed., *Classic Descriptions of Disease* (Springfield, IL: Charles C. Thomas, 1959), 188–90; and "North, Elisha," in *Appletons' Cyclopedia of American Biography, 1600–1889* (New York: D. Appleton and Company, 1888), 4:533–34.

6. Elisha North, *A Treatise on a Malignant Epidemic Commonly Called Spotted Fever* (New York: T. and J. Swords, 1811).

7. A bibliography of works (1768–1902) on cerebrospinal meningitis is available at Cecil Wall, "On Acute Cerebro-Spinal Meningitis Caused by the Diplococcus Intracellularis of Weichselbaum: A Clinical Study," *Medico-Chirurgical Transactions* 86 (1903): 77–79. See also "Epidemic Cerebro-Spinal Meningitis," in William Aitken and Meredith Clymer, *The Science and Practice of Medicine* (Philadelphia, PA: Lindsay and Blakiston, 1868), 445–460; Eduard-Rudolf Müllener, "Six Geneva Physicians on Meningitis," *Journal of the History of Medicine and Allied Sciences* 20, no. 1 (January 1965): 10n30; Lothario Danielson and Elias Mann, "The First American Account of Cerebrospinal Meningitis," *Review of Infectious Diseases* 5, no. 5 (September–October 1983): 969–72; and Alexander Crever Abbott, *The Hygiene of Transmissible Diseases* (Philadelphia, PA: W. B. Saunders, 1899), 119–20.

8. Dr. Lothario Danielson (1765–1841) was born in Hampden County, Massachusetts, as one of the ten children of John Danielson Jr. (1727–1815) and Ruth Blodgett (1728–1807). He, his father, and five

brothers served during the American Revolution. He studied medicine with Dr. Ebenezer Humphrey Phillips (1756–1837) of Charlton, Worcester County, Massachusetts, before opening a practice in Medfield, Norfolk, Massachusetts. He moved to Rochester, Monroe County, New York, in 1826. He moved again to Michigan, where he died in 1841. He married Mary "Polly" Rider (1774–1812) in 1794; their two children died at a young age. He married Hannah Cheney in 1817.

9. Dr. Elias Mann (1778–1807) was born in Medfield, Norfolk County, Massachusetts, as one of the three children of Saban Mann (1747–1800) and Hannah Plimpton (1749–1782). He earned his bachelor's and medical degrees from Harvard College and Harvard Medical College, respectively, in 1800 and in 1805, respectively. He married Keziah Harding (1775–1858) in 1801; they had three children. He died in 1807 at the age of twenty-nine years. Ebenezer Alden, *Early History of the Medical Profession in Norfolk County, Mass.: An Address Delivered before the Norfolk District Medical Society at Its Annual Meeting, May 10, 1853* (Boston, MA: S. K. Whipple and Company, 1853).

10. Lothario Danielson and Elias Mann, "The History of a Singular and Very Mortal Disease Which Lately Made Its Appearance in Medfield," *Medical and Agricultural Register* 1 (1806): 65–69; and Frank J. Grady, "Some Early American Reports on Meningitis," *Journal of the History of Medicine and Allied Sciences* 20, no. 1 (January 1, 1965): 27–32.

11. Dr. François Louis Isidore Valleix (1807–1855) was born in Toulouse, Haute-Garonne, France. As a young man, he moved to Paris to study medicine and serve as an extern in 1829 and as an intern from 1831 to 1833. He received his medical diploma in 1835. He was an ardent disciple of Pierre Charles Alexandre Louis (1787–1872), who developed the numerical method, the forerunner of epidemiology, the modern clinical trial, and evidence-based medicine. While an intern in Parisian hospitals, Dr. Valleix became attracted to the diseases of infancy. In 1838, he turned his attention to the investigation of nervous system diseases. In 1836, he became a physician at the Central Bureau, and beginning in 1841, he served as a physician in the hospitals of Paris. Between 1844 and 1848, he wrote *Guide du Médecin Praticien or Résumé Général de Pathologie Interne et de Thérapeutique Appliqués*, a work in ten volumes, including one (tome IX) on nervous system diseases. He died in 1855 after

contracting diphtheria from a child; he was forty-nine years old. See "M. Valleix" (obituary), *Boston Medical and Surgical Journal* 52 (November 22, 1855): 352–53.

12. F. L. I. Valleix, *Guide Médecin Praticien or Résumé Général de Pathologie Interne et de Thérapeutique Appliqués* (Paris: J. B. Billière, 1847), 6:219.

13. Dr. Meredith Clymer (1816–1902) was born in London, England (while his parents were traveling), as the eldest of the two children of Mary (Marie, Maria) Gratiot (O'Brien) (1790–1853) and George W. Clymer (1785–1848). He was the grandson of George Clymer Sr. (1739–1813), a signer of the American Declaration of Independence on July 20, 1776. Meredith Clymer earned his bachelor's degree from the University of Pennsylvania in 1835 and his medical degree from the University of Pennsylvania School of Medicine in 1837. In 1839, he studied abroad before returning to Philadelphia to practice medicine for ten years, during which time he consulted at the Philadelphia Hospital (1843–1846), served as physician in chief at the Cholera Hospital, and served as a professor of medicine in the Hampden-Sidney College in Richmond, Virginia. He moved to New York City in 1851 to teach the practice of medicine in the ten-year-old Medical Department of the University of the City of New York. He specialized in diseases of the nervous system and the mind. During the American Civil War, he served as a surgeon in the United States Volunteers and as medical director of the Department of the South (1864–1865), which was headquartered on Hilton Head Island, Beaufort County, South Carolina. From 1871 to 1874, he became a professor of mental and nervous diseases at Albany Medical College, Union University, in Albany, Albany County, New York. He authored many medical works, including *The Pathology, Diagnosis and Treatment of Fevers* (1846); *Notes on the Physiology and Pathology of the Nervous System, with Reference to Clinical Medicine* (1868); *Lectures on Palsies and Kindred Disorders* (1870); *Ecstasy and Other Dramatic Disorders of the Nervous System* (1870); *Hereditary Genius* (1870); *Epidemic Cerebro-Spinal Meningitis* (1872), and others. He married Virginia Margaret Garesche (Gareschi) (1827–1849) of Wilmington, Delaware, in 1843 and Eliza "Lily" ("Lillie") Strong Snelling (1838–1922) in 1856. He had no children. He died at home in New York City at the age of eighty-six years. See "Necrology: Meredith Clymer," *Alumni Roster of the University of Pennsylvania* (Philadelphia, PA: University of Pennsylvania General Alumni Society, 1902), 481;

"Death List: Meredith Clymer," *New York Times*, April 21, 1902, 9; and "Obituary, Dr. Meredith Clymer," *British Medical Journal* 1, no. 2159 (May 17, 1902): 1243.

14. Charles Bolduan, "Cerebrospinal Meningitis from the Standpoint of Public Health," *Medical Times* 36, no. 7 (July 1908): 193–195.

15. How to calculate the 8.07 mortality rate:
$782/968,710 = x/10,000$; $x = 8.07$. See Charles Bolduan, "Cerebrospinal Meningitis from the Standpoint of Public Health," *Medical Times* 36, no. 7 (July 1908): 193.

16. Meredith Clymer, *Epidemic Cerebro-Spinal Meningitis* (Philadelphia, PA: Lindsay and Blakiston, 1872), 33.

17. Dr. Robert Koch (1843–1910) was born in Clausthal, a small mining town in Hannover, Niedersachsen (Lower Saxony), Germany, as one of the eighteen children of Hermann Koch (1814–1877), a mining engineer, and Mathilde Julie Henriette Biewend (1819–1871). Robert Koch earned his medical degree from the University of Göttingen (Göttingen, Lower Saxony, Germany) in 1866; worked at a mental hospital in Langenhagen; moved to Niemegk to practice medicine in 1868; moved again in 1869 to Rakwitz, near Posen; and served in the German Army during the Franco-German War in 1870. He next became the district physician in Wollstein (Prussia) in 1872, and he took a position with the Imperial Health Office in Berlin (Prussia) in 1880. On March 24, 1882, he gave his famous address on the discovery of the tubercle bacillus in Berlin. He articulated Koch's Postulates in 1883, became professor of hygiene at the University of Berlin in 1885, opened the Robert Koch Institute for Infectious Diseases in 1900, received the Nobel Prize for his investigations and discoveries in relation to tuberculosis in 1905, and died in 1910. Dr. Koch married Emilie Adolfine Sophie Fraatz (1847–1913) in 1867; they had one child and divorced in 1893. He married Edwig Emma Franziska Freiberg (1872–1945) in 1893. He died of heart disease after being in failing health for a year; he was sixty-seven years old. See Thomas D. Brock, *Robert Koch: A Life in Medicine and Bacteriology* (Berlin: Springer-Verlag, 1988); and "Koch Dies Martyr; Famous Bacteriologist Victim of Exposure in Africa; Discovered Tuberculin; One of World's Leaders in Fight against Consumption; Recipient of Many Honors; Member of Medical Bodies the World Over and Given a Title by the Kaiser," *Evening Star* (Washington, DC), May 28, 1910, 8.

18. *Mycobacterium tuberculosis* resists staining by the Gram stain method of bacterial differentiation devised by the Danish bacteriologist Hans Christian Gram (1853–1938). However, *Mycobacterium tuberculosis* is stainable by a special bacteriological dye (the Ziehl-Neelsen stain) originally developed by Dr. Robert Koch (1843–1910) in 1882 and modified by the bacteriologist Franz Ziehl (1859–1926) in 1882 and 1883 and by the pathologist Friedrich Neelsen (1854–1898) in 1883. See "R. C. Ellis and L. A. Zabrowarny, "Safer Staining Method for Acid Fast Bacilli," *Journal of Clinical Pathology* 46 (1993): 559–560.

19. Dr. Anton Weichselbaum (1845–1920) was born in Schiltern, Krems-Land, Lower Austria, as the son of a barrel maker. He attended the gymnasium in Krems (1855–1863) and studied medicine at the Imperial Medical Surgical Military Hospital and at the University of Vienna, where he earned his medical doctorate in 1869. He subsequently assisted the Bohemian pathologist Dr. Carl Freiherr von Rokitansky (1804–1878) and the Austrian anatomist Dr. Josef Engel (1816–1899) at the University of Vienna. After serving as a military physician, he rose through the ranks at the University of Vienna to become a full professor in 1893 and the rector of the university in 1912. He was among the first physicians to recognize the importance of bacteriology for pathological anatomy and to embrace the science of serology. He trained Dr. Karl Landsteiner (1868–1943), who discovered interagglutination between serum and blood cells, and Dr. Anton Ghon (1866–1936). See K. Cartwright, "Microbiology and Laboratory Diagnosis," *Methods of Molecular Medicine* 67 (2001): 1–8; Anton Weichselbaum, *The Elements of Pathological Histology* (London: Longmans, Green, and Company, 1895); "Anton Weichselbaum," accessed March 3, 2018, http://www.whonamedit.com/doctor.cfm/2874.html; and "Anton Weichselbaum," *Wikipedia*, accessed March 3, 2018, https://en.wikipedia.org/wiki/Anton_Weichselbaum.

20. A Gram-negative bacterium will *not* retain the crystal violet stain used in the Gram-staining method of bacterial differentiation. The Danish bacteriologist Hans Christian Joachim Gram (1853–1938) devised the Gram-staining method in 1884 while he was studying in the laboratory with Carl Friedländer (1847–1887) in Berlin. A few years later, Dr. Carl Weigert (1845–1904) added a final step of staining with safranin, which turned the colorless Gram-negative bacteria red. See Kaivon Madani, "Dr. Hans Christian Joachim

Gram: Inventor of the Gram Stain," *Primary Care Update for OB/ GYNS* 10, no. 5 (September–October 2003): 235–37.

21. Cecil Wall, *On Acute Cerebro-Spinal Meningitis Caused by the Diplococcus Intracellularis of Weichselbaum: A Clinical Study* (London: Royal Medical and Chirurgical Society, 1993), 36–37, 39.

22. Anton Weichselbaum, *Fortschritte der Medicine* 5 (1887), 579, as listed in Cecil Wall, *On Acute Cerebro-Spinal Meningitis Caused by the Diplococcus Intracellularis of Weichselbaum: A Clinical Study* (London: Royal Medical and Chirurgical Society, 1993), 58.

23. Dr. Heinrich Albrecht (1866–1922) was a Viennese bacteriologist who worked under Dr. Anton Weichselbaum. Dr. Albrecht died of tuberculosis at the age of fifty-six years. Dr. Anton Ghon (1866–1936) was an Austrian pathologist and professor in Vienna known for the Ghon complex in pulmonary tuberculosis. He trained under Dr. Karl Landsteiner (1868–1943), who discovered interagglutination between serum and blood cells. See Heinrich Albrecht and Anton Ghon, "About the Etiology and Pathological Anatomy of Meningitis Cerebrospinalis Epidemica," *Vienna Klinische Wochenschrift* 14 (1901): 984–96; and "*Neisseria meningitidis*," in NCBI Taxonomy, *EOL Encyclopedia of Life*, accessed March 3, 2018, http://eol.org/pages/996566/names/synonyms.

24. Charles F. Bolduan, "Cerebrospinal Meningitis from the Standpoint of Public Health," *Medical Times* 36, no. 7 (July 1908): 193–95.

25. Bellevue Hospital, located on acreage between the East River and First Avenue in Manhattan, originated as a separate care area for sick inmates of the City Almshouse in 1735. In 1816, a new Belle Vue [*sic*] almshouse and prison opened near Twenty-Eighth Street and the East River. In 1836, the prisoners housed at Bellevue moved to Blackwell's Island. By 1848, insane patients and paupers were moved out of Belle Vue. Sporadic clinical teaching first took place at Bellevue Hospital in 1804 and increased in 1849 and again in 1857. In 1861, the Bellevue Hospital Medical College opened in a building on the hospital grounds. See Robert Janus Carlisle, *An Account of Bellevue Hospital* (New York: Society of the Alumni of Bellevue Hospital, 1893); Moses King, *King's Handbook of New York 1892* (Boston, MA: Barnes and Noble, 1892), 422–23; Georgina F. Pope, "Bellevue Hospital, Past and Present," *American Journal of Nursing* 5, no. 1 (October 1904): 28–33; and Georgina Pope, "Bellevue Hospital, Past and Present (Concluded)," *American Journal of Nursing* 5, no. 5 (February 1905): 291–96.

26. Dr. Joseph F. McCarthy (1874–1965) was born in Yonkers, Westchester County, New York, as the son of Jeremiah McCarthy and Honorah Moynihan. He attended a local parochial school; worked in a drugstore beginning at the age of fifteen years; earned his pharmacy degree from the New York College of Pharmacy (1896); earned his medical degree from the College of Physicians and Surgeons of New York City (1901); and served as a house staff surgeon Bellevue Hospital (1901–1903) and as an attending physician for a year. He developed cerebrospinal meningitis while serving as an attending physician at Bellevue Hospital. He survived the disease; traveled to the urologic clinics of Berlin, Vienna, and Paris in 1904; and returned to the United States to work at the New York Postgraduate Medical School and Hospital as a professor of urology (1917). He also taught at other medical schools. He developed urologic instruments and surgical procedures and became a renowned urologist. He married Katherine F. Ewald. They had no children. He lived to ninety years of age. See "Joseph Francis McCarthy MD, 1874–1965," William P. Didusch Center for Urologic History, accessed August 15, 2017, http://www.urologichistory.museum/content/collections/uropeople/mccarthy/p1.cfm; and "Joseph Francis McCarthy," accessed August 15, 2017, http://prabook.com/web/person-view.html?profileId=1111777.

27. "Spotted Fever Record: Largest Number of Cases Since Epidemic of 1872," *New York Tribune*, May 12, 1904, 1.

28. Dr. Thomas Darlington (1858–1945) was born in the Williamsburg neighborhood of Brooklyn, New York, as the fourth of the eight children of Thomas Darlington (1826–1903), a sawyer [*sic*], and Hanna Anne Goodliffe (1830–1900). He received his early formal education in the Brooklyn public schools and at Newark High School in Newark, Essex County, New Jersey. He studied science and engineering at the College of the City of New York before earning his medical diploma from the College of Physicians and Surgeons of New York City in 1880. He practiced medicine in Newark, New Jersey (1880–1882); the Kingsbridge neighborhood of the Bronx (1882–1888); Bisbee, Cochise County, Arizona Territory (1888–1891); and then Kingsbridge once again (1891–1904). Mayor George B. McClellan Jr. (served 1904–1909) appointed Dr. Darlington as the New York City health commissioner on January 1, 1904. Dr. Darlington was the first physician to occupy the position. The next mayor, William Jay Gaynor, did not reappoint Dr. Darlington as health commissioner. Dr. Darlington subsequently practiced medicine

and held civic positions (e.g., an appointee to the mayor's committee on sanitation and harbor pollution). He married Josephine Alice Sergeant (1864–1890) in 1886; they had two children. He died at the age of eighty-three years. "Sketches of Appointees: Dr. Thomas Darlington," *New York Tribune*, January 1, 1904, 5; Frances M. Rackemann, "Dr. Thomas Darlington," *Transactions of the American Clinical and Climatological Association* 58 (1946): lvii–lix; and "Thomas Darlington," in Frances E. Quebbeman, *Medicine in Territorial Arizona* (Phoenix, AZ: Arizona Historical Foundation, 1966), 337.

29. "Health Commissioner Darlington Recommends Hot Baths and Sedative Medicine for Scourge of Cerebro-Spinal Meningitis—Disease Not Directly Contagious," *Evening World*, March 18, 1905, 5; "Disease Not Caught from Patient," *New York Tribune*, March 16, 1905, 14; and "Fresh Air for Meningitis: Dr. Darlington Says It Has Proved Better than Serums," *New York Times*, May 6, 1905, 16.

30. Dr. Albert Burns Craig (1867–1905) was born in Auxvasse, Callaway County, Missouri, as the middle child of the nine children of Joseph L. Craig (1832–1926), a farmer, and Mary Elizabeth Jones (1832–1920). Albert Craig moved to eastern Washington to teach school in Spokane, Spokane County, and subsequently served as principal of the Medical Lake Schools in Medical Lake, Spokane County, Washington. He next worked for two years as the steward of the Eastern Washington Hospital for the Insane in Medical Lake under Dr. John McFarland Semple (1857–1932), the asylum superintendent. Albert Craig enrolled in the Jefferson Medical College of Philadelphia in 1897 and graduated as valedictorian of his class of 1901 at the age of thirty-four years. He married Frances Boyd Foster (1880–1925) on October 12, 1904, at her parents' home in Newton, Massachusetts. After the wedding, they moved to Philadelphia, where he succumbed to cerebrospinal meningitis in 1905. At the time of his death, Dr. Craig was assistant editor of *American Medicine* and assistant demonstrator in surgery and anatomy at his alma mater. He was also building a medical practice. See "Dr. Crig [*sic*] Dies a Hero; Former Medical Lake Asylum Steward Victim to Cerebro Spinal Meningitis; Contracted the Disease from Friend—Was Known by Teachers of Eastern Washington," *Evening Statesman* (Walla Walla, Washington), March 25, 1905, 2; "City Will Put Ban on 'Spotted Fever'; Dr. Craig's Death Induces Authorities to Enter upon Strenuous Campaign against Pestilential Cerebrospinal Meningitis,"

Philadelphia Inquirer, March 17, 1905, 1; "Contagion in Horrible Form; Deaths from Cerebrospinal Meningitis; Two Recent Deaths in Philadelphia Have Developed the Medical Theory that the Disease Is Highly Contagious," *Baltimore American* (Baltimore, MD), March 16, 1905, 14; "Doctors Mourn at Craig's Bier; Impressive Funeral Services on Body of Dr. Albert B. Craig, Who Gave Life for a Friend," *Boston Journal* (Boston, MA), March 17, 1905, 3; "Craig's Doctors out of Danger; Those Who Attended Cerebro-Spinal Victim Not Infected; Body of Late Physician Taken to Newton, Mass., after Services in This City," *Philadelphia Inquirer*, March 16, 1905, 16; "Dr. Albert B. Craig, Who Gave His Life in Aiding Friend," *Boston Journal*, March 17, 1905, 3; and "Spotted Fever in Contagion Test; Philadelphia Physicians Watch with Great Interest Persons Exposed through Dr. Craig," *St. Louis Post-Dispatch*, March 22, 1905, 7.

31. See "Plans War on Meningitis. Dr. Darlington Alarmed at Spread—Board Asks Fund for Inquiry," *New York Times*, March 2, 1905, 16; "To Probe Spinal Fever; Health Board Wants Commission to Investigate—Spread Alarming," *New York Tribune*, March 2, 1905, 5; "To Study Meningitis; Dr. Darlington Names Commission Provided for by Board of Estimate," *New York Times*, March 19, 1905, 6; and "79 Spotted Fever Deaths in 2 Months and 18 Days; Dr. Darlington Names Experts—Nature of Cerebro-Spinal Meningitis So Far as Known," *Brooklyn Daily Eagle*, March 18, 1905, 2.

32. The commission members were Dr. Thomas Darlington, Dr. Hermann M. Biggs, Dr. W. K. Draper, Dr. E. K. Dunham, Dr. Simon Flexner, Dr. Walter B. James, Dr. William L. Polk, Dr. William P. Northrup, Dr. Joshua Van Cott, and Dr. W. J. Elser. See Wade W. Oliver, *The Man Who Lived for Tomorrow: A Biography of William Hallock Park, MD* (New York: E. P. Dutton, 1941), 231.

33. Dr. Simon Flexner (1863–1946) was born in Louisville, Jefferson County, Kentucky, as the fourth of the nine children of German immigrants Moritz (Morris) Flexner (1820–1882), a peddler, and Esther Abraham (1835–1905). Simon graduated from the two-year program of lectures at the University of Louisville College of Pharmacy, worked as a druggist, earned a medical diploma from the two-year program of lectures at the University of Louisville Medical Department in 1889, and won a place in the pathology program headed by Dr. William Henry Welch (1850–1934) at the Johns Hopkins University School of Medicine in Baltimore in 1890. In 1892, 1893, and 1899, he studied the cerebrospinal meningitis

epidemic in Maryland, medicine in Europe, and tropical diseases in the Philippines, respectively. He subsequently won a research professorship at the University of Pennsylvania. In 1904, John Davison Rockefeller (1839–1937), the oil magnate and philanthropist, recruited him to direct the fledgling Rockefeller Institute for Medical Research in New York City. When the cerebrospinal meningitis epidemic of 1904 struck New York City, Dr. Flexner embarked on his quest at the Rockefeller Institute to discover a cure for the disease. See James Thomas Flexner, *An American Saga: The Story of Helen Thomas and Simon Flexner* (New York: Fordham University Press, 1993); George Washington Corner, *A History of the Rockefeller Institute, 1901–1953: Origins and Growth* (New York: Rockefeller Institute Press, 1964); and "Rockefeller Money and Medical Science: A Social Investment," in E. Richard Brown, *Rockefeller Medicine Men; Medicine and Capitalism in America* (Berkeley, CA: University of California Press, 1979), 105–11. For images of the Rockefeller Institute Laboratory in 1912, visit Rockefeller University's "Founder's Hall and the Hospital" web page, accessed March 3, 2018, http://digitalcommons.rockefeller. edu/hospital-of-institute/15/ngs. For images of Dr. Simon Flexner, visit the National Library of Medicine web page, accessed March 3, 2018, https://collections.nlm.nih.gov/?utf8=%E2%9C%93&PID=n lm%3Anlmuid-56431240R-bk&q=flexner.

34. John Davison Rockefeller Sr. (1839–1937) was born in Richford, Tioga County, New York, as the second child and the eldest son of William Avery Rockefeller (1810–1906), a peddler, and Eliza Davison (1813–1889). The family moved frequently before settling in Cleveland, Cuyahoga County, Ohio, where John D. Rockefeller became a bookkeeper at age sixteen (1855), an oil refiner at age twenty (1859), and a founder of Standard Oil Company in 1870. As a philanthropist, he provided the funds to found the University of Chicago in 1890 and the Rockefeller Institute for Medical Research in Manhattan in 1901. See Ron Chernow, *Titan: The Life of John D. Rockefeller Sr.* (New York: Vintage, 1984); and George Washington Corner, *A History of the Rockefeller Institute, 1901–1953: Origins and Growth* (New York: Rockefeller Institute Press, 1964).

35. Dr. Hermann Michael Biggs (1859–1923) was born in Trumansburg, Tompkins County, New York, as the younger of the two sons of Joseph Hunt Biggs (1827–1877), a hardware merchant, and Melissa A. Biggs (1826–1910). He attended Cornell University in Ithaca

(1879–1882) and earned his medical degree from Bellevue Hospital Medical College in 1883. In 1892, he joined the New York City Health Department, where he remained a driving force for the rest of his life. See C.-E. A. Winslow, *The Life of Hermann M. Biggs, Physician and Statesman of the Public Health* (Philadelphia, PA: Lea and Febiger, 1929).

36. For a brief history of the New York City Board of Health, see Charles F. Bolduan, "Over a Century of Health Administration in New York City," *Department of Health of the City of New York Monograph Series* 13 (March 1916), 23–24; and Arthur Bushel, *Chronology of New York City Department of Health (and Its Predecessor Agencies) 1655–1966* (New York: New York City Health Department, March 1966), accessed April 3, 2018, https://www1.nyc.gov/assets/doh/downloads/pdf/history/chronology-1966centennial.pdf.

37. The Research Laboratory of the New York City Board of Health originated as the Diagnostic Bacteriological Laboratory of the New York City Board of Health on May 4, 1893. The Diagnostic Bacteriological Laboratory was the first public health diagnostic bacteriological laboratory in the United States. Dr. Hermann Biggs (1859–1923), chief of the newly created New York City Board of Health Division of Pathology, Bacteriology, and Disinfection, founded the laboratory to assist the city in the diagnosis of diphtheria. Dr. William Hallock Park (1863–1939), the "bacteriological diagnostician of diphtheria," directed the laboratory in the Laboratory and Division Office of the New York City Board of Health at 42 Bleecker Street in Lower Manhattan. The laboratory soon commanded larger laboratory space in the Criminal Court Building at 100 Centre Street in Lower Manhattan. The number of bacteriologists and technicians employed for the laboratory examinations of diphtheria and tuberculosis specimens increased to twelve to handle the volume of incoming specimens designated for culture. On December 23, 1894, the New York City Board of Health received funds to manufacture diphtheria antitoxin. The first antitoxin, manufactured by Dr. Park and Dr. Anna Williams (1863–1954), was available on January 1, 1895. The New York City Board of Health provided the antitoxin free of charge to private physicians in New York City. Private physicians could obtain the antitoxin at culture stations organized by Dr. Park to collect swabs for culture from the throats of patients. In February 1895, the staff of the Division of Pathology, Bacteriology, and Disinfection expanded to include an assistant

pathologist, an assistant chemist, four assistant bacteriologists, several additional laboratory assistants, and a collector of culture tubes. In October 1895, Dr. Park and his staff moved from the Criminal Court Building to the second floor of the Willard Parker Hospital Disinfecting Station on the west side of Willard Parker Hospital, located on East Sixteenth Street, Manhattan, near the East River. The Diagnostic Bacteriological Laboratory next became known as the Hospital Laboratory. In 1905, the Hospital Laboratory moved out of the Willard Parker Hospital Disinfecting Station into a new six-story building called the Laboratory Building. It was located on the east side of Willard Parker Hospital, nearer to the nearby East River. The Hospital Laboratory and the Laboratory Building subsequently became known as the Research Laboratory (also Research Laboratories). Dr. Park directed the Research Laboratory and the municipal production of all vaccines, antitoxins, and sera for use by the physicians and patients of New York City. He sold surplus antitoxin to other cities to raise funds to support the work of the Research Laboratory. In 1908, the New York City municipal government purchased acreage in Otisville, Orange County, New York, to erect a municipal tuberculosis sanatorium. In 1909, it gave some of the acreage to the Research Laboratory to build facilities for stabling the horses and other animals used in the manufacture of sera, antitoxins, and vaccines. See "The Function of Research in Municipal Health Administration," *Monthly Bulletin of the Department of Health of the City of New York* 1, no. 3 (March 1911): 51–53; Hermann M. Biggs, "The Development of the Research Laboratories," *Monthly Bulletin of the Department of Health of the City of New York* 1, no. 3 (March 1911): 54–56; C.-E. A. Winslow, *The Life of Hermann M. Biggs, Physician and Statesman of the Public Health* (Philadelphia, PA: Lea and Febiger, 1929); Wade W. Oliver, *The Man Who Lived for Tomorrow: A Biography of William Hallock Park, MD* (New York: E. P. Dutton, 1941); Hermann M. Biggs, *Brief History of the Campaign against Tuberculosis in New York City: Catalogue of the Tuberculosis Exhibit of the Department of Health, City of New York, 1908* (New York: Department of Health, 1908), 12–13; and Ben Freedman, "The First State Board of Health Laboratories in the United States," *Public Health Reports* 69, no. 9 (September 1954): 868.

38. See Simon Flexner, "Experimental Cerebrospinal Meningitis and Its Serum Treatment," *Journal of the American Medical Association* 47,

no. 8 (August 25, 1906): 560–66; and Simon Flexner, "Experimental Cerebro-Spinal Meningitis in Monkeys," *Journal of Experimental Medicine* 9, no. 2 (March 14, 1907): 142–67.

39. Dr. Charles Frederick Bolduan (1873–1950) was born in Bielefeld, North Rhine-Westphalia, Germany, to William Bolduan and Juliane Caroline Dreibholz. In 1879, he immigrated to the United States. He attended Brooklyn public schools, returned to Germany to earn a pharmacy doctorate in Berlin, returned to the United States, became a naturalized citizen in 1894, earned a medical degree from the College of Physicians and Surgeons of New York City in 1901, and joined the New York City Board of Health in 1904. He organized the New York City Board of Education's Bureau of Education in 1914 and directed it for decades. From 1918 to 1928, he worked for the United States Public Health Service. In 1906, he married Adele Jonsson; they had one child. His second wife was Herma Engelsdorff, whom he married in 1928. He died in Bellevue Hospital at the age of seventy-seven years. See John Shrady, *The College of Physicians and Surgeons, New York: A History* (New York: Lewis Publishing Company, 1903), 2:529; and "Dr. C. F. Bolduan, Health Official," *Brooklyn Daily Eagle*, July 5, 1950, 15.

40. "Quarantine for Meningitis; New York Health Official Thinks the Disease Is Communicable," *Democrat and Chronicle* (Rochester, New York), April 22, 1905, 2; and Wade W. Oliver, *The Man Who Lived for Tomorrow: A Biography of William Hallock Park, MD* (New York: E. P. Dutton, 1941), 232.

41. Centers for Disease Control and Prevention, "Measures of Risk," Principles of Epidemiology in Public Health Practice, Third Edition, accessed August 12, 2018, https://www.cdc.gov/ophss/csels/dsepd/ ss1978/lesson3/section2.html.

42. Simon Flexner, "Experimental Cerebrospinal Meningitis and Its Serum Treatment," *Journal of the American Medical Association* 47, no. 8 (August 25, 1906): 560–66.

43. Wade W. Oliver, *The Man Who Lived for Tomorrow: A Biography of William Hallock Park, MD* (New York: E. P. Dutton, 1941), 300.

44. Simon Flexner, "Experimental Cerebrospinal Meningitis and Its Serum Treatment," *Journal of the American Medical Association* 47, no. 8 (August 25, 1906): 560–66.

45. Wilhelm Kolle and August Wasserman, "Versuch zur Gewinnung und Wertbestimmung eines Meningococcenserums," *Deutsch Medizinische Wochenschrift* 32 (1906): 609–12.

46. Gustaf Jochmann, "Versuche zur Serodiagnostic und Serotherapie der epidemischen Genickstarre," *Deutsch Medizinische Wochenschrift* 32 (1906): 788–93.

47. Simon Flexner and James Wesley Jobling, "Serum Treatment of Epidemic Cerebro-Spinal Meningitis," *Journal of Experimental Medicine* 10, no. 1 (January 1, 1908): 194–95; and Thomas Lynch, "Cerebrospinal Meningitis Treatment," *Medical Herald* 31, no. 6 (June 1912): 297–98.

48. Dr. William Hallock Park (1863–1939) was born at 164 West Eleventh Street, Manhattan, as one of the three sons of Rufus Park (1813–1896), a merchant, and Hannah Joanna Hallock (1835–1881). Rufus Park had been widowed twice before marrying Hanna Hallock and had three children by his previous wives, including one daughter, Julia, with whom William was close throughout his life. William H. Park attended the Boys' Public School on West Thirteenth Street, and in 1883, at the age of twenty years, he completed the five-year combined secondary-collegiate program at the College of the City of New York. He earned his medical degree from the College of Physicians and Surgeons of New York City in 1886; performed postgraduate work at Roosevelt Hospital in New York City (1886–1889), advancing through the ranks to become house surgeon; studied medicine in Europe for a year; returned to New York City to run a private medical practice for a year; and joined the staff of Dr. T. Mitchell Prudden's laboratory (1890–1892) at the College of Physicians and Surgeons of New York City to study diphtheria. At the same time, he was associated with Bellevue Hospital, the Vanderbilt Clinic of the College of Physicians and Surgeons, Roosevelt Hospital, and Manhattan Eye and Ear Hospital as a laryngologist. In 1892, Dr. Park published his first scientific paper describing his method of diagnosing diphtheria by demonstrating diphtheria bacilli in cultures. In 1893, Dr. Hermann Biggs recruited him as the "bacteriological diagnostician of diphtheria" of the New York City Board of Health's Diagnostic Bacteriological Laboratory. Dr. Park steadily advanced to become director of the Research Laboratory of the New York City Board of Health. He never married and had no children. He died suddenly of heart disease in 1939 at the age of seventy-six years. He had worked for the New York City Board of Health for forty-three years. See William H. Park and Alfred Beebe, "Diphtheria and Allied Pseudo-Membranous Inflammations, a Clinical and Bacteriological Study," *Medical Record* 42 (July 30 and August 6, 1892): 113–25,

141–47; Wade W. Oliver, *The Man Who Lived for Tomorrow: A Biography of William Hallock Park, MD* (New York: E. P. Dutton, 1941); Page Cooper, *The Bellevue Story* (New York: Thomas Y. Crowell Company, 1948), 135–43; Harry Filmore Dowling, "Field, Ward, and Laboratory: Where the Infectious Disease Physician Worked," *Journal of Infectious Diseases* 153, no. 3 (March 1986): 390–96; "Dr. William Park, Health Official," *Brooklyn Daily Eagle,* April 6, 1949, 15; and Hans Zinsser, "William Hallock Park, 1863–1939," *Journal of Bacteriology* 38, no. 1 (July 1939): v-3–3.

49. August Wassermann, "Über die Bisherigen Erfahrungen mit dem Meningococcen-Heilserum bei Genickstarre-kranken," *Deutsch Medizinische Wochenschrift* 33 (1907): 1585–87.

50. Georg Jochmann, "Versuche zur Serodiagnostik und Serotherapie der epidemischen Genickstarre," *Deutsche Medizinische Wochenschrift* 1, no. 1 (1906): 788–93. See also Wade W. Oliver, *The Man Who Lived for Tomorrow: A Biography of William Hallock Park, MD* (New York: E. P. Dutton, 1941), 303; and Abraham Sophian, *Epidemic Cerebrospinal Meningitis* (St. Louis, MO: C. V. Mosby Company, 1913), 175.

51. Simon Flexner, "Experimental Cerebrospinal Meningitis and Its Serum Treatment," *Journal of the American Medical Association* 47, no. 8 (August 25, 1906): 566.

52. Simon Flexner and James Wesley Jobling, "Serum Treatment of Epidemic Cerebro-Spinal Meningitis," *Journal of Experimental Medicine* 10, no. 1 (January 1, 1908): 141–203.

53. Ibid., 196.

54. Ibid., 202.

55. Dr. Heinrich Ireneaus Quincke (1842–1922), a German internist and pathologist, invented the spinal needle (Quincke needle) in 1891 to perform lumbar, or spinal, puncture to relieve the pressure resulting from hydrocephalus and to provide cerebrospinal fluid for bacterial diagnosis and culture. See Heinrich Quincke, "Die Lumbalpunktion des Hydrocephalus," *Verhandl Kong Innere Medizinisch Wiesbaden* 10 (1891): 321–31; and Heinrich Quincke, "Über Lumbalpunktion," *Berliner Klinische Wochesnschrift* 32 (1895): 861–62, 929–33. The earliest American print articles on lumbar puncture include George W. Jacoby, "Lumbar Puncture of the Subarachnoid Space," *New York Medical Journal* 62 (December 28, 1895): 813–18; Lewis A. Conner, "The Technique of Lumbar Puncture," *New York Medical Journal* 71 (May 12, 1900): 723–25; Alfred Hand Jr., "A Critical

Summary of the Literature on the Diagnostic and Therapeutic Value of Lumbar Puncture," *American Journal of the Medical Sciences* 120 (October 1900): 463–69; Henry Heiman, "The Technics of Lumbar Puncture in Children: With Particular Reference to the Pressure of the Cerebrospinal Fluid," *Mount Sinai Hospital Reports* 5 (1905–1906): 114–23; and Samuel Joseph Kopetzky, "Lumbar Puncture: A General Review of Its Value and Applicability," *American Journal of the Medical Sciences* 131 (April 1906): 648–74.

56. The cerebrospinal fluid space is the area surrounding, bathing, and nourishing the spinal cord. The spinal cord is a long, thin bundle of nervous tissue and support cells that extends from the medulla oblongata of the brainstem to the lumbar region. The cerebrospinal fluid space is also known as the subarachnoid space, which lies between the arachnoid mater and the pia mater, two of the coverings of the spinal cord (the pia is closest to the spinal cord itself, the arachnoid is the next outer layer, and the dura is the outermost layer). The cerebrospinal fluid space is also known as the thecal sac and the membranous tube of dura mater. Two terms commonly used to describe the administration of medication directly into the cerebrospinal fluid space are *intraspinal* (within the spinal column) and *intrathecal* (within the theca).

57. Missouri Census Data Center, Missouri State Library, Jefferson City, Missouri, accessed May 19, 2018, http://mcdc.missouri.edu/trends/historical.shtml.

58. "Many Cases of Meningitis; Kansas City Physicians Say It's Almost an Epidemic; Death Has Come Quickly in a Majority of Cases—Doctors Expect the Coming of Balmy Weather Will Stop Its Spread," *Kansas City Star*, April 10, 1899, 2.

59. "The Meningitis Epidemic; The Coming of Warmer Weather Seems Not to Have Checked It," *Kansas City Star*, April 14, 1899, 16.

60. Dr. Edwin Taylor Phillips (1860–1921) was born in Albion, Iowa. He earned his medical degree from the Kansas City Medical College and the Kansas City College of Physicians and Surgeons in 1883. After practicing medicine in Kansas City for almost forty years, he developed influenza and moved to San Diego, where he died at the age of sixty-one. He married Nettie A. Morrison (1866–1895) in 1885 in Kansas City; she died in Chicago in 1895. They had no children. "Death of Dr. E. T. Phillips: Word Is Received of Physician's End in California," *Kansas City Star*, September 30, 1921, 6; "Mrs. Nettie Phillips's Death; Husband Unexpectedly Called in Chicago

by a Telegram Announcing It," *Kansas City Star*, November 13, 1895, 1; and "Dr. Edwin Taylor Phillips," in Arthur Wayne Hafner, *Directory of Deceased American Physicians, 1804–1929* (Chicago, IL: American Medical Association, c. 1993).

CHAPTER 1

A HOSPITAL AND HEALTH BOARD FOR KANSAS CITY, 1908-1911

In 1908, the hospital and health department scene in Kansas City was undergoing rapid change. On Tuesday, August 4, 1908, Kansas City voters approved a new city charter[1-2] that established the Kansas City Board of Hospital and Health[3] (also known as the Board of Hospital and Health of Kansas City, Missouri) to oversee, among its varied responsibilities, the Kansas City Hospital and Health Department. The three names—the Kansas City Board of Hospital and Health, the Kansas City Hospital and Health Department, and the Hospital and Health Board of Kansas City—were interchangeable in common parlance after implementation of the new city charter in 1908. In that same year, Kansas City's mayor, Thomas Theodore Crittenden Jr.,[4] appointed the following three members to the new board: Charles Watson Armour,[5] head of the Armour Packing Company in Kansas City, Kansas; Edward Fletcher Swinney, president of the First National Bank of Kansas City; and William Perry Motley,[6] an insurance executive originally from Tuskegee, Macon County, Alabama.

On Friday, September 14, 1908, the Hospital and Health Board of Kansas City appointed Dr. Walter Sewell Wheeler[7] as Kansas City health commissioner and executive officer of the Hospital and Health Board of Kansas City.[8] Dr. Wheeler graduated from the

State Normal School at Warrensburg, Johnson County, Missouri, and Jefferson Medical College in Philadelphia. After moving to Kansas City, he served as the inspector of contagious diseases from 1901 to 1903 while conducting a successful medical practice.[7] As the new health commissioner, Dr. Wheeler initially received a salary of $2,400 per year. He was forbidden from practicing medicine while serving as health commissioner.[8]

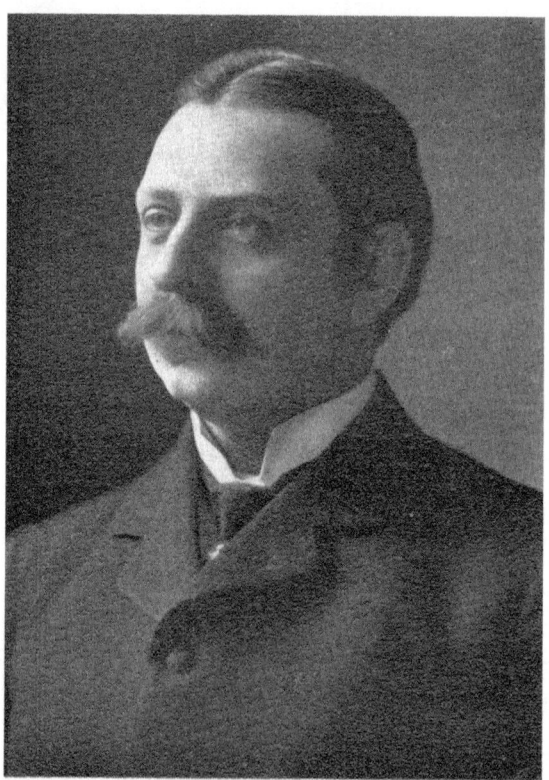

Dr. Charles Sewell Wheeler (1858–1918), 1904. The photographer is unknown. The image was scanned from "Wheeler, Walter Sewell, Class of 1885," in George M. Gould (ed.), *The Jefferson Medical College of Philadelphia, 1826–1904; A History* (New York: Lewis Publishing Company, 1904), 2:274.

The Hospital and Health Board of Kansas City—henceforth the Hospital and Health Board—and its new health commissioner next began searching for a physician superintendent to manage the newly erected Kansas City General Hospital, a hallowed municipal institution dating to 1869.[9] In 1903, the Kansas City City [sic] Council issued $225,000 in bonds to build a new five-hundred-bed Kansas City General Hospital to replace the overcrowded two-hundred-bed Kansas City Municipal Hospital. Philanthropist Thomas Hunton Swope[10] donated four and a half acres atop a hill in midtown Kansas City on which to build the new general hospital. The completed hospital would eventually occupy the block bounded by Locust Street, Kenwood Avenue, Twenty-Third Street, and Twenty-Fourth Street in Kansas City. Construction began in 1905.

In the fall of 1908, the center and north buildings of the Kansas City General Hospital were ready for occupancy. The center and north buildings were four stories above the raised basement and subbasement. The center building's main facade and entrance faced west onto Locust Street high above the Kansas River. Above the entrance was a gigantic, decorative white ornamental stone panel etched with the following words from Shakespeare's play *The Merchant of Venice*: "The quality of mercy is not strain'd / It droppeth as the gentle rain from heaven."[11] A long north–south corridor connected the center building to the north building in each of the four stories. Doors at the ends of these corridors could be closed to disconnect each floor of each building, rendering it a unit or small hospital unto itself. Hardwood covered eight-inch-thick concrete floors. An east–west corridor ran the entire length of the upper floors of the north building, which contained the patient wards. Each ward contained dressing rooms, quiet rooms, and toilet facilities. The hospital morgue was in the basement of the north building. The center building contained the main operating room on the fourth floor, the administrative offices, and other facilities.[12] The Hospital and Health Board met in the administrative offices of the center building. The nearby old Kansas City Municipal Hospital was not torn down. Instead, it became Kansas City General Hospital No. 2, also known as the Old Hospital and as the Old Hospital for Negroes.[13]

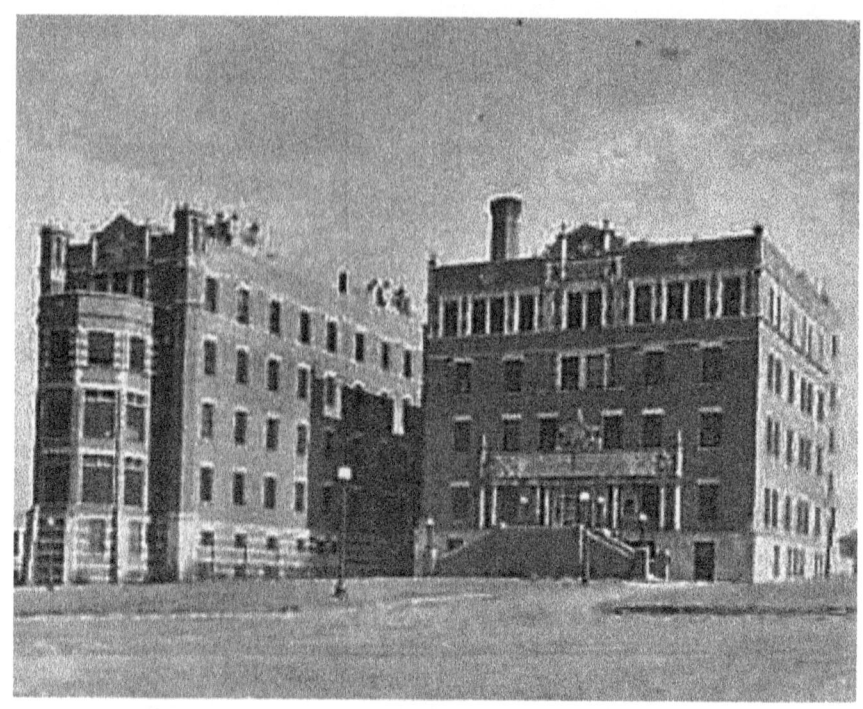

The administration building and north wing of the Kansas City General Hospital, circa 1908. The south wing has not yet been completed. Courtesy of the Missouri Valley Collections, Kansas City, Missouri. The photographer is unknown.

As time passed, the Hospital and Health Board and Dr. Wheeler were unable to identify a suitable candidate for the position of superintendent. Finally, they appointed the hospital house surgeon, thirty-four-year-old Dr. James Park Neal,[14] as the acting superintendent. Dr. Neal, previously the school superintendent of the public schools of Daviess County, Missouri, only recently had graduated from medical school in Kansas City. Other Hospital and Health Board appointees[15] included Dr. George Pierce Pipkin[16] to head the Old Hospital, Dr. Frank Johnson Hall[17] to head the department of food inspection, Dr. Murry (Murray) Stone[18] to head the hospital pathology department, and Miss Harriet Leck[19] to serve as the superintendent of the Kansas City General Hospital nurses and, in 1910, also as the superintendent of the (Kansas City) General Hospital Training School for Nurses.[20-21]

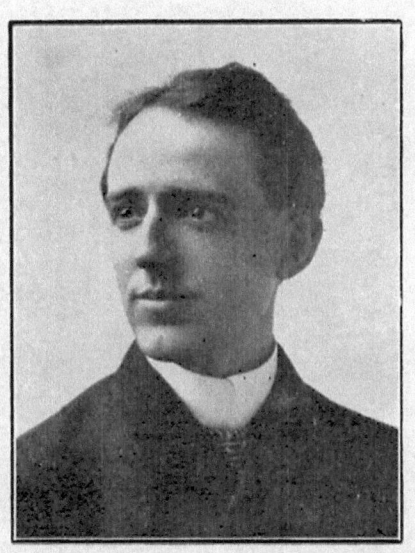

FRANK JOHNSON HALL.
M. D., 1897, (Kansas City Medical College).
Associate Professor of Clinical Pathology, and
Director of the Pathological Laboratory, 1905.

Dr. Frank Johnson Hall (1875–1946), 1907. The image was scanned from *The Jayhawker* (yearbook), University of Kansas, 1907, p. 16. The image is courtesy of the Kenneth Spencer Research Library, University of Kanas Libraries, University of Kansas, Lawrence, Kansas.

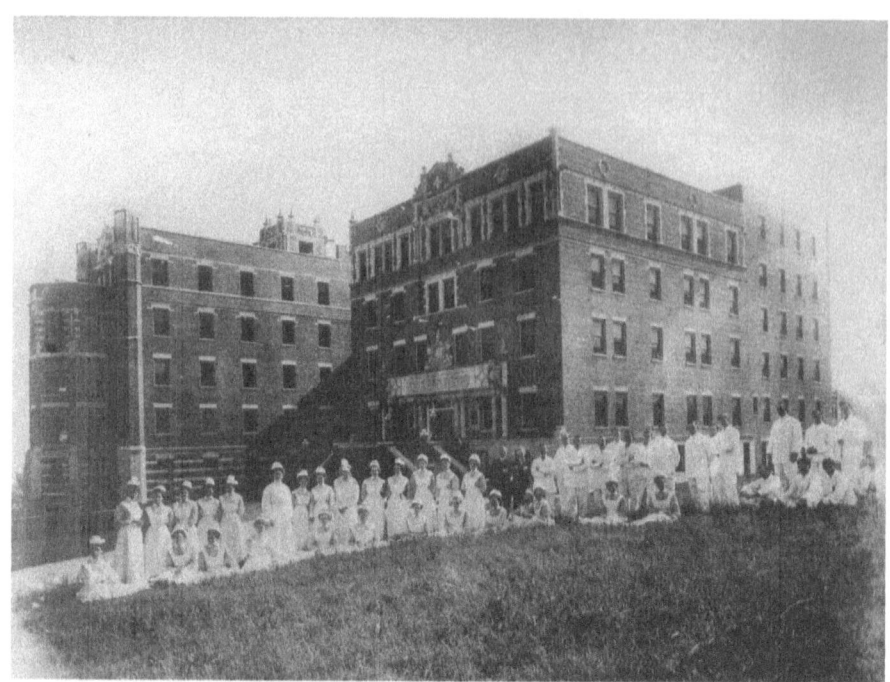

The students nurses standing with Miss Leck (in the center of the
nursing group, wearing all white) in front of the center and north
buildings of the Kansas City General Hospital, circa 1912. Kansas
City General Hospital interns and two unidentified men in suits
are on the right side of the group photo. The image is courtesy
of the Truman Medical Center Archives, Kansas City, Mo.

One of the first challenges met by Dr. Neal, Dr. Pipkin, and
Miss Leck was to transfer sixty-nine patients from the Old Hospital
into the north building of the Kansas City General Hospital on
October 8, 1908.[22] Some fifty-eight African American patients
remained in the main building of the Old Hospital, while white
patients with tuberculosis and other contagious diseases remained
in an isolation annex of the Old Hospital.

In mid-1909, the Hospital and Health Board published its first
monthly data on the occurrence of common contagious diseases
in Kansas City for the time interval of September 1, 1908, to
April 30, 1909.[23] In the inaugural year of contagious-diseases
data collection (1908–1909), data collection was intermittent and
incomplete. Nevertheless, the Hospital and Health Board received

reports of 298 cases of diphtheria, 239 cases of scarlet fever, 135 cases of measles, 18 cases of whooping cough, 98 cases of typhoid fever, 108 cases of chickenpox, 54 cases of pneumonia, 13 cases of mumps, 36 cases of smallpox, and 46 cases of tuberculosis.[23] After reviewing the data, Dr. Wheeler crowed, "I am pleased to report to this Honorable Board that the city has been practically free from all contagious maladies during the past year [1908–1909]. This in part is due to the fact that the city is reasonably clean, and to the diligent work on the part of Charitable Institutions and Sanitary Inspectors."[24]

Of note, the Hospital and Health Board received no reports of cerebrospinal-meningitis cases during the inaugural year of data collection (1908–1909).[25] The reason, said Dr. Wheeler, was that cerebrospinal meningitis was unknown in Kansas City previous to January 1, 1911; therefore, its reporting was not required.[25] Dr. Wheeler was wrong about the occurrence of cerebrospinal meningitis in Kansas City. As noted in the introduction to this book, the disease made an appearance during the cold months of 1898 to 1899. In addition, the *Kansas City Star*[26] reported three deaths from meningitis in 1908,[27] of which one was further specified as "spinal meningitis."[28] Many physicians did not identify the type of meningitis during the early years of data collection because to do so required examination of cerebrospinal fluid. Acquisition of cerebrospinal fluid from a patient required knowledge of the technique of performing a lumbar puncture procedure and microscopy, both of which were in their infancies in clinical medicine.

On Wednesday, August 4, 1909, the Hospital and Health Board hired[29] Dr. George Wilse Robinson[30] to succeed Dr. Neal as the superintendent of the Kansas City General Hospital. Dr. Robinson previously had served as superintendent of the State Hospital for the Insane (No. 3) in Nevada, Vernon County, Missouri (1905–1907). His salary as superintendent of the Kansas City General Hospital was $3,600 per year.[31]

On Tuesday, February 1, 1910, a new vital-statistics reporting law resulting from the passage of the Revised Statutes of the State of Missouri in 1909[32-33] went into effect statewide. The State Board of Health of Missouri, located in Jefferson City (which had a population of twelve thousand in 1910[34]), the capital of Missouri, appointed 912 vital-statistics registrars, which it apportioned among the 114 counties of the state. These registrars were responsible for producing monthly reports of births, deaths (including the cause of death), and cases of reportable contagious diseases.[35] The new statute included provisions for certain penalties for data-reporting noncompliance.[35] The 912 vital statistics registrars sent their data to Dr. Frank Baker Hiller,[36] the state vital-statistics registrar and the secretary of the State Board of Health of Missouri. The health department officials of large Missouri cities, such as St. Louis and Kansas City, had been collecting citywide birth and death data for two years, but now they were subject to the provisions of the new state law, which meant reporting their data to the state registrar on the blank forms provided by the latter, as well as other requirements.

The prevalence of meningitis in Kansas City between April 1909 and April 1910 was barely measurable, with a report of only one case of meningitis (etiology not specified) at the Kansas City General Hospital.[37] In addition, no Kansas City newspapers reported cases of, or deaths from, meningitis in Kansas City between April 20, 1909, and April 19, 1910.[38-39]

On Wednesday, June 15, 1910, Dr. George Wilse Robinson, for unknown reasons, resigned as superintendent of the Kansas City General Hospital after having served only ten months. One of his achievements was to publicize in medical schools around the country the availability of intern positions at the Kansas City General Hospital. When he started his job, he observed the paucity of interns, which he said handicapped the work of the hospital. He screened prospective interns by means of a competitive examination. Of one hundred applicants, he selected eighteen, among whom were graduates from Rush Medical College in Chicago, Illinois, and the medical schools associated with the Johns Hopkins University, the University of Pennsylvania, Northwestern University, McGill University, Washington University, St. Louis

University, Texas University, and the University of Virginia. The interns served for one year, from July 1 to June 30 of the following year. They received no salary. Dr. Robinson wrote, "It is to be hoped that [the interns] will find this service so profitable and pleasant that there will be no difficulty in securing an adequate number of interns of the best quality in the future."[40]

A month passed. On Wednesday, July 20, 1910, the Hospital and Health Board successfully recruited[41] Dr. Louis Willard Luscher[42] to succeed Dr. Robinson as superintendent of the Kansas City General Hospital. Dr. Luscher was a veteran Kansas City physician who had served as a military surgeon in armies around the world. One of his first worries as superintendent of the Kansas City General Hospital was the lack of a proper contagious-diseases hospital. In 1910, patients with contagious diseases were still housed in an annex to the Old Hospital. Dr. Luscher lobbied the municipal government for a new contagious-diseases hospital close by the Kansas City General Hospital.

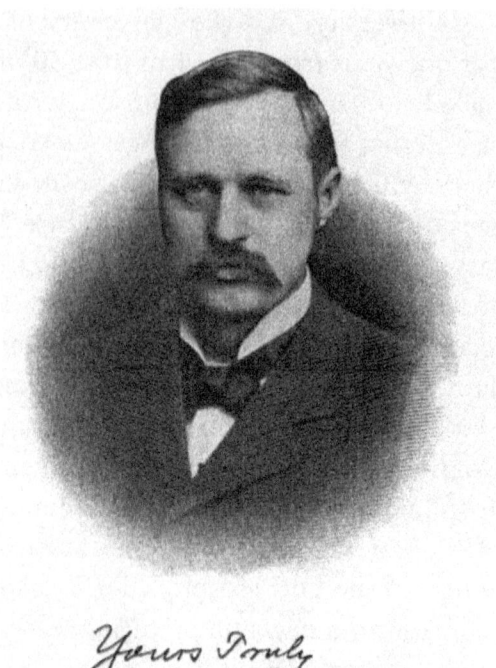

Dr. Louis Willard Luscher (1858–1922), 1904. The artist is unknown. The image was retrieved from "Luscher, Louis Willard," in Howard Louis Conard (ed.), *Encyclopedia of the History of Missouri: A Compendium of History* (New York: Southern History Company, 1901), 4:135–136.

Six months passed. Between late January 1911 and February 13, 1911, four unnamed children developed cerebrospinal meningitis in Kansas City,[43] astounding their unnamed private physicians. An unknown person or persons urgently requested antimeningitis serum from Dr. Flexner in New York City. Two of the children died before the serum arrived, but the two others apparently benefitted from the serum.[43] The Kansas City newspaper report of this first use of Flexner antimeningitis serum in Kansas City was subdued compared to the spirited report of the serum's first use three years earlier in the municipal hospital of St. Louis, Missouri (January 1908).[44] St. Louis physicians adopted advances in cerebrospinal meningitis therapy more quickly than did their counterparts in Kansas City.

In mid-March 1911, cerebrospinal meningitis struck a fifth Kansas City child: four-year-old William Joseph Barbeau Jr., a celebrity's son. On Sunday, April 2, 1911, William succumbed to the disease at St. Joseph (St. Joseph's) Hospital[45] in Kansas City.[46] The nature of his treatment, if any, is unknown. His father was William Joseph "Jap" Barbeau (1882–1969), a Major League Baseball third baseman who was playing for the St. Louis Cardinals at the time of his young son's death.[47] The five pediatric cerebrospinal meningitis cases within six weeks (late January through March 1911) placed the medical and health department communities on edge.

One week later, on Sunday, April 9, 1911, the Kansas City General Hospital admitted its first cerebrospinal meningitis patient: an adult named Mr. Michael Givens. Railroad authorities had found him unconscious on a Missouri Pacific Railway train that had stopped in Kansas City on its way from New York City to Pueblo, Colorado. Hospital physicians performed a lumbar puncture procedure, withdrew cerebrospinal fluid, examined it under a microscope, and diagnosed cerebrospinal meningitis based on the presence of meningococci. The hospital physicians infused an amount of Flexner antimeningitis serum equal to the amount they had withdrawn.[48] Mr. Givens improved rapidly and apparently recovered. Mr. Givens's case was the first known time that Kansas City General Hospital physicians had used Flexner antimeningitis serum (April 9, 1911).

Monday, April 17, 1911, was the last day of the fiscal year 1910–1911 for the Hospital and Health Board. Staff soon began work on the board's third annual report. It contained no data on the occurrence of meningitis in the city because meningitis still was not a reportable disease, as noted above. However, Dr. Luscher, as superintendent of the Kansas City General Hospital, tracked all of the hospital's medical diseases and, hence, monitored the occurrence of cases of meningitis. Dr. Luscher reported only one case of cerebrospinal meningitis—presumably Mr. Givens—who had been admitted to the Kansas City General Hospital between April 18, 1910, and April 17, 1911.[49] The six known cerebrospinal meningitis cases (i.e., the one known case of cerebrospinal meningitis admitted to the Kansas City General Hospital and the five pediatric cases cared for in their homes) during the data-collection period of April 1910 to April 1911 suggests a low prevalence of the disease for the time interval.[50]

Another month passed. On Thursday, May 4, 1911, a *Kansas City Star* article ran an anonymous article praising antimeningitis serum for its role in reducing the proportion of individuals who died of their cerebrospinal meningitis. The article read, "From an average of 80 deaths from cerebrospinal meningitis out of 100 cases, the proportion has been changed to an average of only 20 deaths out of 100 cases. The decrease in the number of deaths is the result of the use of an antitoxin serum, and latter figures are based only on cases where the serum was used. Not only are many more lives saved, but where the serum is used the physical vigor of the person affected is more likely to be restored." It added that as of May 4, 1911, the Kansas City General Hospital physicians had treated six afflicted patients with Flexner antimeningitis serum, and of the six afflicted patients, only one had died.[51] This new information suggested that the Kansas City General Hospital had admitted five more patients with cerebrospinal meningitis after Mr. Givens (i.e., between April 9, 1911, and May 4, 1911).

Just as cases of cerebrospinal meningitis were beginning to show up in Kansas City in January through May of 1911, the Rockefeller Institute for Medical Research announced its discontinuation of free Flexner antimeningitis serum to health department officials and private physicians in the United States and abroad. The institute cited two reasons. First, Dr. Flexner believed he had validated the efficacy and safety of the serum in humans with cerebrospinal meningitis. Second, the institute wanted to move the funds dedicated to antimeningitis serum research, manufacture, and distribution to other lines of investigation.[52] The institute had been the only place to obtain the serum in the United States since early 1908, when Dr. Flexner offered it free of charge to physicians. Who would produce the antimeningitis serum after the exit of the institute from the marketplace?

The Rockefeller Institute for Medical Research suggested that municipal and state public health department officials and commercial pharmaceutical companies were the appropriate venues for the routine preparation of the serum for general use. As these venues ramped up to produce antimeningitis serum, the meningitis division of the Research Laboratory of the New York City Board of Health agreed to produce and distribute the serum at a minimal cost. The Research Laboratory was experienced in the manufacture of antimeningitis serum. Recall that Dr. Park, the director of the Research Laboratory, had sent the laboratory's own antimeningitis serum to Hartford, Connecticut, physicians in 1905, as noted above. Dr. Park's head of the meningitis division of the Research Laboratory in 1911 was twenty-six-year-old Dr. Abraham Sophian.[53] To ease the transition from the manufacture of antimeningitis serum by the Rockefeller Institute for Medical Research to its manufacture by the Research Laboratory, Dr. Flexner presented the Research Laboratory Meningitis Division with the Rockefeller Institute's two antimeningitis-serum-producing horses.[54]

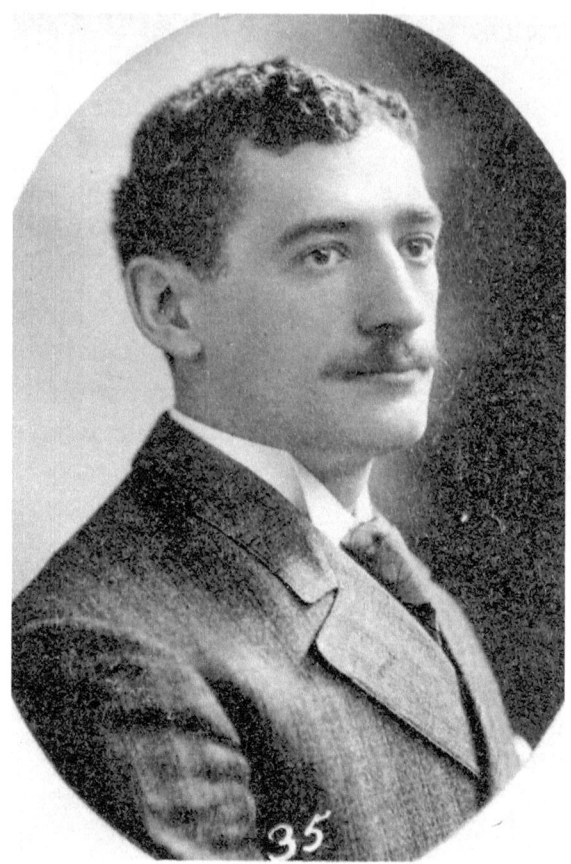

Dr. Abraham Sophian (1885–1957), 1906, aged twenty-one years at his graduation from Cornell University Medical College in New York City. This image is from the class composite held by the Weill Cornell Medicine Samuel J. Wood Library, New York City. Courtesy of Medical Center Archives of New York-Presbyterian/Weill Cornell.

The first commercial pharmaceutical company to enter the antimeningitis serum market was the H. K. Mulford Company, which was headquartered in Philadelphia. The company, founded in the late 1880s by pharmacist Henry Kendall Mulford,[55-56] had produced the first commercial diphtheria antitoxin in the United States in 1895.[57] Mr. Mulford tipped his hat to Dr. Park at the Research Laboratory for providing the knowledge to manufacture antimeningitis serum.[58]

In early July 1911, a representative of H. K. Mulford Company submitted to Dr. Hiller, the secretary of the State Board of Health of Missouri, as noted above, a proposal to provide low-cost antimeningitis serum to Missouri counties. At the Saturday, July 15, 1911, meeting of the State Board of Health of Missouri, Dr. Hiller presented the proposal.[59] The board members present—Drs. Ernest Franklin Robinson[60] (president), Milton Pleam Overholser,[61] and Louis Edward Bunte[62]—did not act on the proposition.[63] Soon after, the H. K. Mulford Company opened a branch office at 915 Broadway, Kansas City.[64]

During the same State Board of Health of Missouri meeting on Saturday, July 15, 1911, Dr. Hiller introduced a resolution to specify the exact "infectious, contagious, or communicable diseases" deemed dangerous to the public health by the State Board of Health of Missouri. The Revised Statues of Missouri of 1909 had specified the creation of the list, but the board had not yet created the list. The diseases deemed "infectious, contagious, or communicable and dangerous to the public health" by the State Board of Health of Missouri on July 15, 1911, were "anthrax, Asiatic cholera, bubonic plague, *cerebrospinal meningitis* [emphasis added], diphtheria (membranous croup), erysipelas, glanders, hydrophobia, infantile paralysis, leprosy, pellagra, pneumonia, pulmonary or laryngeal tuberculosis, scarlet fever, smallpox, tetanus, typhoid fever, typhus fever, whooping cough, and yellow fever."[65] The State Board of Health of Missouri required the vital-statistics registrars throughout the state of Missouri to begin tracking and reporting these diseases monthly on Monday, January 1, 1912.[23] The Kansas City health department officials complied with the new rule on reporting the list of infectious, contagious, or communicable diseases beginning January 1, 1912.

A third item of action during the meeting of the State Board of Health of Missouri on July 15, 1911, was the approval of certain rules applicable to the processing of contagious-diseases corpses. For example, the new rules said that corpse preparation for burial must occur in the room or house where the death occurred, disposition by cremation or burial must occur immediately, and only those persons absolutely necessary to assist could attend the disposition of the body. The new board rules governing the processing of contagious-diseases corpses also forbade public funerals over the remains of those dying from the specified diseases.[65]

Also, in July 1911, Dr. Luscher welcomed a new group of interns to the Kansas City General Hospital. Dr. Luscher expressed gratitude to his predecessor, Dr. Robinson, for establishing a worthy internship program at the hospital.[66] The new group of interns soon to be sorely tested included Dr. Arthur Hawley Parmelee (schooled at Rush Medical College, Chicago, Illinois),[67] Dr. Harry Johnson Schott (Rush Medical College),[68] Dr. Frederick Worley Aves (University of Texas Medical Branch at Galveston),[69] Dr. Frank Randall Teachenor (University of Kansas Medical School),[70] Dr. Benjamin Weems Turner (University of Texas Medical Branch at Galveston),[71] Dr. Richard William Spicer Sr. (University of Pennsylvania School of Medicine),[72] and Dr. Elmer Vail Eyman (Rush Medical College).[73] The interns ranged in age from twenty-three to twenty-eight years.

Eight members of the attending medical staff who taught and oversaw the work of this special group of interns were Dr. Franklin E. Murphy (University of Pennsylvania School of Medicine),[74] Dr. Hugh D. Hamilton (Missouri Medical College and the McDowell Medical College, St. Louis),[75] Dr. John Lincoln Robinson (University Medical College of Kansas City and the College of Physicians and Surgeons of New York City),[76] Dr. Frederick McKendrie Lowe (Rush Medical College),[77] Dr. Charles Clinton Conover (University Medical College of Kansas City),[78] and Dr. Scott Parker Child (University of Pennsylvania School of Medicine).[79] Drs. Robinson, Lowe, and Conover served as attending physicians from Friday, September 1, 1911, to Friday, March 1, 1912, and Drs. Murphy, Hamilton, and Child served as attending physicians from Friday, March 1, 1912, to Sunday, September 1, 1912.[80]

On Sunday, August 13, 1911, the Kansas City government awarded a contract for the construction of a new contagious-diseases hospital (also called the contagion hospital or the isolation hospital) to replace the isolation annex of the Old Hospital. The site for the new contagious-diseases hospital was several hundred feet north of the north building of the Kansas City General Hospital, on the southeast corner of Twenty-Third Street and Robert Gilham Road. The cost was $75,000.[81]

The new contagious-diseases hospital consisted of two three-story buildings with separate entrances and a one-story structure connector between them. The connector building functioned as a receiving and detention ward. When the diagnosis of a disease was uncertain, physicians could lodge patients in the connector until the disease sufficiently developed to make a diagnosis. The ground floor of each building was designed for the care of patients with mild contagious diseases. The second and third floors of each building were reserved for the care of patients with moderate to severe contagious diseases. Patients with measles, diphtheria, scarlet fever, meningitis, and smallpox were to receive their care in the new contagious-diseases hospital.[82] The planned opening of the contagious-diseases hospital was Wednesday, January 1, 1913.[83] Dr. Luscher hoped there would be no major epidemic during the cold months of late 1911 and early 1912.

On Monday, October 30, 1911, Dr. Frank Hall reminded his fellow Kansas City physicians to obtain a supply of antimeningitis serum in case they encountered a patient with cerebrospinal meningitis during the upcoming cold months.[84] Did they listen to his advice?

CHAPTER 1 NOTES

1. The unabridged city charter of 1908 is available at Rees Turpin, George King, and Charles L. Shannon, *Charter and Revised Ordinances of Kansas City, 1909* (Kansas City, MO: Frank T. Riley Publishing Company, 1909).

2. For more information on the Kansas City Charter of 1908, see "The New Charter," *Kansas City Medical Index-Lancet* 31, no. 346 (October 1908): 370–71; Roy Ellis, *A Civic History of Kansas City, Missouri* (Springfield, MO: Press of Elkins-Swyers Company, 1930), 171–87; and "What the New Charter Is; The Changes in City Government Explained in Simple Language; From Other Municipalities Ideas Were Taken and Compiled into One Document—the Civil Service Idea Goes into Effect with the New Administration," *Kansas City Star* (Kansas City, MO), February 18, 1910, 12.

3. Rees Turpin, George King, and Charles L. Shannon, *Charter and Revised Ordinances of Kansas City, 1909* (Kansas City, MO: Frank T. Riley Publishing Company, 1909), 444–50.

4. Thomas Theodore Crittenden Jr. (1863–1938) was born near Springfield in Sangamon County, Illinois, as one of the four children of Caroline Wheeler "Carrie" Jackson (1839–1917) and Thomas Theodore Crittenden Sr. (1832–1909), the governor of Missouri (1881–1885). Governor Crittenden was perhaps best known for ridding Missouri of Jesse James (1882) and other Missouri outlaws. The family moved to Warrensburg, Johnson County, Missouri, where young Thomas Jr. spent his boyhood. He graduated from the public schools of that city and from Missouri State University in 1883, moved to Kansas City in 1884, and entered the real estate business. He was appointed as the deputy clerk of the Missouri Court of Appeals, Western District, in Kansas City. He was the Democratic nominee for county clerk in 1894 and won the election. He was renominated and elected to the same position in 1898. He was elected mayor of Kansas City and served from 1908 to 1910. He declined to run again. He returned to his real estate and investment business for the duration of his life. He married Jennie Mason Rogers in 1888; they had two children. He died of bronchopneumonia at the age of seventy-four years. See "Making Kansas City, Missouri Great! The Reforms of Mayor Thomas T. Crittenden Jr. Has Made Kansas City a Model—Every Campaign Promise Made Good,"

Plaindealer (Topeka, KS), April 16, 1909, 1; and "T. T. Crittenden Rites," *Kansas City Star*, August 1, 1938, 5.

5. Charles W. Armour's term as president expired on April 20, 1909. William P. Motley succeeded Mr. Armour as president of the board. See Hospital and Health Board, *First Annual Report of the Board of Hospital and Health of Kansas City, Missouri, for Fiscal Year April 20, 1908, to April 19, 1909, Inclusive* (Kansas City, MO: Kansas City Board of Hospital and Health, 1909), front pages; and Edwin D. Shutt, "The Saga of the Armour Family in Kansas City, 1870–1900," *Heritage of the Great Plains* 23 (Fall 1900): 25–41.

6. William Perry Motley (1858–1938) was born in Tuskegee, Macon, Alabama, as one of the six children of John Glenn Motley (1823–1908), a minister, and Louisa Perry (1830–1908). He married Sallie Willis Carpenter (1862–1939) in 1887 in Kansas City; they had no children. He worked as an agent for the Pacific Mutual Insurance Company and served as head of the Hospital and Health Board for many years. "W. Perry Motley Dies; Former Hospital and Health Board Head Ill since June; About Ten Years Ago He Had Retired from the Life Insurance Business—Known Widely as a Fisherman," *Kansas City Star*, February 6, 1938, 11.

7. Dr. Walter Sewell Wheeler (1858–1918) was born in Winchester, Frederick County, Virginia, as the eldest of the four children of John Cummings Wheeler (1831–1908), a farmer and a bugler during the American Civil War, and Katharine "Kate" Copenhaver (1837–1903). Young Walter moved with his parents to Sedalia, Pettis County, Missouri, and, from there, to Knobnoster, Johnson County, Missouri. He received his early formal education in private schools in Missouri; graduated from the State Normal School at Warrensburg, Johnson County, Missouri, in 1880; and entered a preparatory course at the University of Missouri while teaching school in Johnson County, Missouri, for two years. He next enrolled at Jefferson Medical College in Philadelphia, Pennsylvania, in 1882, where he earned his medical degree in 1885. Following graduation, he returned to Missouri; practiced medicine with Dr. F. P. Claycomb at Moundville, Vernon County, Missouri, for three years; and moved to Kansas City to practice medicine. He served as the surgeon to the Kansas City Jail (1893–1895); the chief deputy coroner for Kansas City and Jackson County (1896–1900); and the vice president (1890–1891) and president of the Jackson County Medical Society (1891–1892). He taught courses at local medical, dental, and pharmacy schools;

served as a consulting physician at the German Hospital in Kansas City; and worked as the inspector of contagious diseases for Kansas City during the administration of Mayor J. A. Reed (1901–1903). He was the first health commissioner of Kansas City (1908–1915), serving through four different mayoral administrations. He resigned because of complaints of his carrying on a large private practice, which was forbidden of health commissioners. He married Frances "Frankie" A. Miller (1858–1950) in 1896; they had no children. He died at home at the age of sixty years. See "Wheeler, Walter Sewell, Class of 1885," in George M. Gould, ed., *The Jefferson Medical College of Philadelphia, 1826–1904; A History: Benefactors, Alumni, Hospital, Etc.; Its Founders, Officers, Instructors* (New York: Lewis Publishing Company, 1904), 2:274–75; "Dr. W. S. Wheeler Gets a Place; He Is Appointed Investigating Physician for the [State] Health Board," *Kansas City Star*, November 11, 1901, 1; "Dr. Wheeler Will Quit," *Kansas City Star*, February 22, 1915, 6; "Dr. William S. Wheeler Dies; Former Health Department Head a Physician Here for Thirty Years," *Kansas City Star*, April 24, 1914, 4.

8. "Health Office to Wheeler; Appointments of the New Board Announced This Morning; The New Head of the Department Is an Expert on Contagious Diseases—The Names of Those Chosen for Other Positions," *Kansas City Star*, September 14, 1908, 2.

9. The Kansas City Municipal Hospital, a charitable institution under municipal control, opened in 1870 as a fifteen-bed, one-story wood-frame structure at Twenty-Second and McCoy Streets in Kansas City. The wood-frame building burned down in 1874. In 1875, two wood-frame structures, one each for female and male patients, replaced the burned-down building. In 1880, a Kansas City ordinance created the first Kansas City Board of Health, which oversaw the administration of city hospitals, the prevention and control of contagious diseases, the collection of vital statistics, sanitation, and the inspection of foods and dairies. In 1884, the city erected a brick hospital building to accommodate forty patients. This building, along with the two wood-frame buildings, served as the City Hospital until 1895. In 1895, the city demolished one wood-frame structure and replaced it with a two-story brick building that contained the administrative offices, a ward for the insane, a women's ward, and a surgical department. The City Hospital now consisted of two brick buildings and a single wood-frame structure. The wood-frame building—St. George's

Hospital (Pest House)—housed patients with contagious diseases. In 1897, the city remodeled the two-story brick building and erected in its rear a clinical amphitheater with seats for 150 medical students. In 1899, after St. George's Hospital burned down, the city erected a one-story, forty-four-bed brick building for patients with contagious diseases. By 1899, Kansas City boasted three brick hospital buildings with 175 beds. In 1903, the hospital expanded its number of beds to two hundred by placing cots in its hallways. The medical profession of Kansas City lobbied the business community to raise funds to erect a new city hospital. In 1903, Kansas City citizens voted bonds of $225,000 to pay for the new city hospital to be built at Twenty-Third and Cherry Streets. See Carrie Westlake Whitney, *Kansas City Missouri, Its History and Its People, 1800–1908* (Chicago, IL: S. J. Clarke Publishing Company, 1908), 1:477–78; John Punton, "Hospitals of Kansas City," in D. M. Bone, *Kansas City Annual, 1907* (Kansas City, MO: Bishop Press, 1906), 61–64; "History of the Kansas City General Hospital," *Jackson County Medical Journal* 26 (October 1, 1932): 11–25; "Kansas City General Hospital," *Historic American Building Survey*, National Park Service, HABS NO. MO-251, accessed April 8, 2018, https://cdn.loc.gov/master/pnp/habshaer/mo/mo0500/mo0513/data/mo0513data.pdf; Barbara M. Gorman, Richard D. McKinzie, and Theodore A. Wilson, *From Shamans to Specialist: A History of Medicine and Health Care in Jackson County, Missouri* (Kansas City, MO: Jackson County Medical Society, 1981), 72, 78, 79; and "General Hospital: Not Just Soap Opera; Old Building Saw Both High Jinks, Misery," *Kansas City Times*, July 1, 1985, 13.

10. Thomas Hunton Swope (1827–1909) was born in Stanford, Lincoln County, Kentucky, as the eldest of the seven children of John Brevett Swope (1799–1881) and Frances Ann Hunton (1804–1847). He graduated from Central University in Kentucky in 1848 and took his senior year at Yale College, earning his bachelor's degree in 1849. After graduation, he studied medicine but did not earn a degree. He lived in Nashville, Davidson County, Tennessee (1849–1852), and in New York City (1852–1853) before exploring the mineral regions of Georgia and East Tennessee (1854). He then entered real estate in Missouri, where he lived first in St. Louis and then in Kansas City. In 1864, he invested in mines in Colorado, Arizona, and Montana. He later sold most of his interest in these mines and purchased more real estate in Kansas City. He eventually became the largest individual

landowner in Kansas City. Later in life, he began to donate his real estate holdings (e.g., to Park College in Missouri and Central University in Kentucky) and the four-and-a-half-acre site for the construction of the new Kansas City General Hospital in 1905. He died unexpectedly at age eighty-one under mysterious circumstances, which led to the famous murder trial of Dr. Bennett Clark Hyde, the Swope family physician and the husband of one of Mr. Swope's nieces. Mr. Swope never married and had no children. See "Thomas Hunton Swope," in *Supplementary History of the Yale Class of 1853* (New Haven, CT: Tuttle, Morehouse, and Taylor, 1894), 339; "Thomas Hunton Swope," in *Catalogue of the Officers and Graduates of Yale University, 1701–1910* (New Haven, CT: Tuttle, Morehouse, and Taylor, 1910), 1173–74; Giles Fowler, *Deaths on Pleasant Street* (Kirksville, MO: Truman State University Press, 2009); and "Dr. Hyde and Mr. Swope," KC History, Missouri Valley Special Collections, Kansas City Public Library, accessed May 19, 2018, http://www.kchistory.org/week-kansas-city-history/dr-hyde-and-mr-swope.

11. "The quality of mercy" is a quote by Portia in act 4, scene 1 of William Shakespeare's late-sixteenth-century play *The Merchant of Venice*. The scene is set in a Venetian court of justice, where Portia is begging Shylock, a Venetian Jewish moneylender, for mercy. Williams Shakespeare, *The Merchant of Venice* (Cambridge, England: Cambridge University Press, 2018).

12. John Punton, "Hospitals of Kansas City," in D. M. Bone, *Kansas City Annual, 1907* (Kansas City, MO: Bishop Press, 1906 [*sic*]), 61–64; and "Kansas City General Hospital, Photographs, Historic and Descriptive Data," Historic American Building Survey, National Park Service, Rocky Mountain Regional Office, Denver, Colorado, HABS No. MO-251, accessed July 28, 2017, https://cdn.loc.gov/master/pnp/habshaer/mo/mo0500/mo0513/data/mo0513data.pdf.

13. Samuel U. Rodgers, "Kansas City General Hospital No. 2, A Historical Summary," *Journal of the National Medical Association* 54, no. 5 (September 1962): 525–639; and "Old Hospital for Negroes; The Health Board Decides to Segregate the City's Patients," *Kansas City Star*, November 1, 1908, 12.

14. Dr. James Park Neal (1874–1941) was born in Smyth County, Virginia, as one of the approximately ten children of Joseph Marion Neal (1845–1923) and March Virginia Humphrey (1851–1929). He moved with his family to Jamesport, Daviess County, Missouri, as

a young boy. He taught grammar in the Jamesport schools before becoming the school commissioner of Daviess County in 1901. He married Imogene O. Briggs (1879–1957) in 1902 and moved to Kansas City in 1904. It is unknown at present where James Park Neal earned his medical diploma in Kansas City. He died of a stroke at St. Joseph Hospital, where he had served as a surgeon for three decades. He and Imogene had no children. See "Dr. J. Park Neal Is Dead; Cerebral Hemorrhage Is Fatal to Surgeon, 67; First Superintendent of the General Hospital Had Practiced Here Thirty-Three Years—Native of Jamesport," *Kansas City Star*, December 12, 1941, 31.

15. Hospital and Health Board, *First Annual Report of the Board of Hospital and Health of Kansas City, Missouri, for Fiscal Year April 20, 1908, to April 19, 1909, Inclusive* (Kansas City, MO: Kansas City Board of Hospital and Health, 1909), 36, 52.

16. Dr. George Pierce Pipkin (1870–1922) was born in Glenville, Nevada County, Arkansas, as the son of Dr. James Andrew Pipkin (1846–1915) and Elizabeth Bernice Johnston (1845–1893). He earned his bachelor's degree from the University of Texas in Austin in 1896 and received his medical degree from the University of Texas Medical Branch at Galveston in 1898. He performed postgraduate work at the University of Chicago. He was the assistant city physician in Kansas City in 1903. He served as superintendent of the Kansas City General Hospital No. 2 beginning in 1908 and as the superintendent of the Kansas City General Hospital from 1915 to 1917. He moved to Lancaster, Dallas County, Texas, around 1917 and died from complications following an appendectomy in 1922 at the age of fifty-two years. He married Ruth Adaline Moody (1875–1963) in 1900; they had four children. "No Hospital Changes Now; The Board Says the Phthisis Sanitarium Will Have to Be Built; Where the Leeds Farm Receives the Tubercular Patients, Negroes Will Go in the New Building," *Kansas City Star*, February 1, 1909, 1; "Lancaster Physician Dies in Dallas after Operation," *Dallas Morning News*, October 15, 1922, 5; and "George P. Pipkin," in Arthur Wayne Hafner, *Directory of Deceased American Physicians, 1804–1929* (Chicago, IL: American Medical Association, c. 1993).

17. Dr. Frank Johnson Hall (1875–1946) was born on a farm near Liberty, Clay County, Missouri, as the only child of Allan Reed Hall (1851–1889), a cattleman, and Theodora (Dora) Johnson (born in 1858), the daughter of Dr. Francis Marion Johnson (1835–1893).

Frank Hall grew up on the family's Liberty farm and on a cattle ranch in Oklahoma before moving to Kansas City after his father's death in 1889. His mother married William E. Wilson (born in 1857), a grocer, in 1898; they had no children. Frank Hall graduated from Garfield Grade School in Kansas City in 1892; Central High School in Kansas City in 1897; and the Kansas City Medical College, which existed from 1881 to 1905, in 1900. He performed postgraduate work at the University of Chicago in 1901, 1902, and 1903. He served as a consultant pathologist at the Kansas City General Hospital and founded the American Biologic Company, which held a license to propagate the rabies virus vaccine after the method of Pasteur for use in preventing rabies in exposed humans during the virus's incubation period. Dr. Frank Hall also gained national fame during the murder trial of Dr. Bennett Clark Hyde, the alleged murderer of Thomas H. Swope (1827–1909), the Kansas City notable and philanthropist who donated the land for the new Kansas City General Hospital in 1905. Dr. Hall also served as the Kansas City–based pathology department editor for the newly reorganized *Medical Herald* beginning in November 1911. Dr. Hall married Mary Eleanor Whitney (1881–1952) in 1898; they had eight children. He retired in 1943 and died three years later at the age of seventy-one years. See "Dr. Frank Hall Dies; Pathologist Here 46 Years Was 71; Retirement in 1913 Follows Active Career in Medical Profession—A Member of Many Groups," *Kansas City Star*, February 25, 1946, 12; "More Victories over Death; A Serum Reduces the Proportion of Fatal Meningitis," *Kansas City Star*, May 4, 1911, 3; and "Meningitis Serum Used Here; Dr. Frank Hall Says the Flexner Treatment Is Not New Here," *Kansas City Star*, October 30, 1911, 5. For more information on Dr. Hall's involvement in the Swope trial, see Giles Fowler, *Deaths on Pleasant Street* (Kirksville, MO: Truman State University Press, 2009), 79–81, 102, 135–36; "How Did Swope Die; A Medical Examination Made of the Body of the Millionaire," *Kansas City Star*, January 14, 1910, 1; "'Give the Barber Glasses'; How a Kansas City Physician Used Sherlock Holmes Methods," *Kansas City Star*, January 17, 1910, 2; "One Grain! Dr. Hektoen Says 1/6th Grain of Strychnine Was Found in Col. Swope's Liver; Strychnine Injected: Nurse Testifies Dr. Hyde Ordered Hypodermics after Convulsions Began; Dr. Hektoen Is Called; The Chicago Chemist Tells of the Analysis Which Showed the Presence of Strychnine," *Kansas City Star*, February 8, 1910, 1;

"Dr. Frank Hall Testifies: The Tonic Could Not Have Caused the Death, the Physician Says," *Kansas City Star*, February 9, 1910, 12; "At the Hypothetical Stage; Lawyer in the Hyde Trial Begun Practice for Scientists Yesterday," *Kansas City Star*, April 30, 1910, 2; and "Dr. Hyde Arrested as Swope's Slayer; Accused of First Degree Murder, He Has Hearing and Is Released on Bail," *New York Times*, February 11, 1910, 1.

18. Dr. Murry (Murray) Chaffee Stone (1880–1951) was born in Leominster, Worcester County, Massachusetts, as one of the two sons of Charles Prescott Stone (1847–1905) and Ella Linette Aldrich (1851–1940). He earned his medical degree from Harvard Medical School in 1903. He practiced medicine while serving as the pathologist at Burbank Hospital in Fitchburg, Worcester County, Massachusetts (1903–1910), before moving west to Kansas City to become the pathologist of the Kansas City General Hospital for eighteen months. Next, he moved to Jefferson City, Cole County, Missouri (1912–1914), to work as the state bacteriologist for the State Board of Health of Missouri. He finally settled in Springfield, Greene County, Missouri, where he opened a clinical pathology laboratory and served as the county coroner. He married Eleanor Mabel Taft (1881–1969) in Fitchburg, Massachusetts, in 1906; they had three children and divorced in 1924. He married Elizabeth Tuck (1906–1989) in 1937; they had one child. Dr. Stone was a charter member of the American Society of Clinical Pathologists. He died of complications from gallbladder disease at the age of seventy-one years. Jonathan Fairbanks and Clyde Edwin Tuck, *Past and Present of Green County: Early and Recent History and Genealogical Records of Many of the Representative Citizens* (La Crosse, WI: Brookhaven Press, 2012).

19. Miss Harriet Leck (1878–1962) was born in Middle Musquodoboit, Halifax County, Nova Scotia, Canada, as one of the seven children of Henry John Leck (1846–1902), a farmer, and Ellen McLeod (1844–1924). The family left Canada to settle in Owatonna, Steele County, Minnesota, around 1895. In 1902, at the age of twenty-four years, Miss Leck trained at the nurses' training school associated with Scarritt Hospital in Kansas City. She joined the nursing staff at the Kansas City General Hospital in 1908 and subsequently served as the superintendent of nurses (1908–1914) and as the superintendent of the (Kansas City) General Hospital Training School for Nurses (1910–1914). She then moved to Detroit, Wayne County, Michigan,

to work as the principal of the Grace Hospital Training School for Nurses. In 1920, she moved to New Haven, New Haven County, Connecticut, to become president of the Visiting Nurse Association there. The same year, she was joined by a daughter, Harriet Ruth Leck. In 1931, at the age of fifty-three years, she married Daniel Lawrence Rourke (1878–1955), the secretary of the Rourke-Eno Paper Company. She died at the age of eighty-five years. "Mrs. Harriet L. Rourke," *Hartford Courant* (Hartford, CT), August 18, 1962, 4; and Harriet Leck, "The Helen Newberry Nurses' Home," *Modern Hospital* 10 (January to June 1918): 264–66. An image of Miss Leck is available in an advertisement titled "The General Hospital a School for Nurses, Colored Department," in *Crisis, A Record of the Darker Races* 9, no. 2 (December 1914): 56.

20. The Kansas City Municipal Hospital superintendent established a training school for nurses in 1902 under a city ordinance that promoted the training of women as professional nurses. On October 9, 1908, the training school came under the direct control of the Hospital and Health Board, and on March 2, 1909, it updated its name to the "General Hospital Training School for Nurses, Kansas City, Mo." The nurses resided in the nurses' apartment on the fourth floor of the north building of the hospital. Their instruction included general care of the sick, making beds, changing bed and body linen, managing helpless patients in bed, giving baths, keeping patients warm or cool, preventing or dressing bed sores, and properly managing patients under various conditions with different diseases. See Hospital and Health Board, *Second Annual Report of the Board of Hospital and Health of Kansas City, Missouri, for Fiscal Year April 20, 1909, to April 19, 1910, Inclusive* (Kansas City, MO: Kansas City Board of Hospital and Health, 1910), 27, 39; and "A Three-Year Term for Student Nurses," *Kansas City Star*, July 20, 1910, 1.

21. A complete list of the medical and surgical staff appointed to serve in the Kansas City General Hospital from September 1908 to June 1, 1909, is available in the Hospital and Health Board of Kansas City, *First Annual Report of the Board of Hospital and Health of Kansas City, Missouri, for Fiscal Year April 20, 1908, to April 19, 1909, Inclusive* (Kansas City, MO: Kansas City Board of Hospital and Health, 1909), front pages.

22. "Ill, Yes, but So Different; The City's Sick Are in Their New Home Now," *Kansas City Star*, October 8, 1908, 8; "No Trouble to Move

the Sick," *Kansas City Star*, October 9, 1908, 12; "Moving into the Hospital; The New City Institution to Be Formally Opened Next Week," *Kansas City Star*, September 19, 1908, 9; "Kansas City's New General Hospital," *Kansas City Star*, September 20, 1908, 1.

23. Hospital and Health Board, *First Annual Report of the Board of Hospital and Health of Kansas City, Missouri, for Fiscal Year April 20, 1908, to April 19, 1909, Inclusive* (Kansas City, MO: Kansas City Board of Hospital and Health, 1909), 52.

24. Ibid., 36.

25. Dr. Wheeler's full comment follows: "Previous to January 1, 1912, the reporting of cases of meningitis to the health department was not required, and previous to January 1, 1911, epidemic meningitis was an unknown disease to this community." "Report on Meningitis," Hospital and Health Board, *Fourth Annual Report of the Hospital and Health Board, for Fiscal Year April 17, 1911, to April 15, 1912, Inclusive* (Kansas City, MO: Hospital and Health Board, 1912), 55.

26. The *Kansas City Star*, originally named the *Kansas City Evening Star*, was founded in 1880 by William Rockhill Nelson (1841–1915) and Samuel E. Morss (1852–1903). Its morning competitors were the *Kansas City Times* and the *Journal*. In 1901, Mr. Nelson purchased the *Kansas City Times* and its morning Associated Press franchise. See "Our History," *Kansas City Star*, accessed May 19, 2018, http://www.kansascity.com/customer-service/about-us/.

27. "Brief Bits of City News," *Kansas City Star*, January 10, 1908, 15; "Brief Bits of City News," *Kansas City Star*, January 31, 1908, 10; and "Happenings of the City," *Kansas City Star*, October 9, 1908, 7.

28. "Brief Bits of City News," *Kansas City Star*, January 31, 1908, 10.

29. "Dr. G. Wilse Robinson Appointed Superintendent by the Board; The Former Chief of the State Hospital at Nevada Will Take Charge August 15—Dr. J. Park Neal Has Been Retained," *Kansas City Star*, August 4, 1909, 11.

30. Dr. George Wilse Robinson (1871–1958) was born in Appleton City, Missouri, as one of the six children of George Woodson Robinson (1844–1931), a farmer, and Cornelia Robinson (1843–1926). He grew up on a farm near Appleton City; graduated from Beaumont Medical College, which existed from 1890 to 1903, in St. Louis, Missouri; practiced medicine in Joplin, Missouri, for four years; and moved to Kansas City in 1902 to found a neurological hospital. He left Kansas City for the Nevada State Hospital, where he served as superintendent for two years (1905–1907) before returning to

Kansas City. He served as superintendent of the Kansas City General Hospital for eighteen months (1909–1910). See "Veteran Doctor Succumbs at 86; Dr. George Wilse Robinson, Formerly Headed Missouri Medical Association," *Joplin Globe* (Joplin, MO), January 23, 1958, 3; and "Nevada State Hospital," Kirkbride Buildings, accessed April 8, 2018, http://www.kirkbridebuildings.com/buildings/nevada/.

31. "A Hospital Job in the Balance; Health Board May Not Appoint Another House Surgeon at the General," *Kansas City Star*, January 13, 1910, 7.

32. "New Law to Go into Effect; Vital Statistics Law Begins February 1," *Marshall Republican* (Marshall, MO), January 21, 1910, 2; "New Law in Effect; That Pertaining to Vital Statistics in Missouri," *Sedalia Democrat* (Sedalia, MO), February 1, 1910, 7; "Health Board Names 900 Doctors to Make Reports; They Will Help Carry Out Provisions of the New Vital Statistics Law," *St. Louis Post-Dispatch*, January 15, 1910, 3.

33. See *Revised Statutes of the State of Missouri, 1909* (Jefferson City, MO: Hugh Stephens Printing Company, 1910).

34. See "Historical Population," in "Jefferson City, Missouri," *Wikipedia*, accessed May 6, 2018, https://en.wikipedia.org/wiki/Jefferson_City,_Missouri.

35. See "Article II, Registration of Births and Deaths; Health, Public, and Vital Statistics," Section 6651, Chapter 53, *Revised Statutes of the State of Missouri, 1909* (Jefferson City, MO: Hugh Stephens Printing Company, 1910), 2:2114–24.

36. Dr. Frank Baker Hiller (1869–1934) was born in Iowa as one of the two children of Royal M. Hiller (1842–1915), a store clerk and notary republic, and Edmoria (Eddie) S. Crampton (1846–1886). He grew up in small towns in Clark County, Missouri, the most northeastern county in the state. His mother died when he was seventeen years old. He earned his medical degree from Rush Medical College in Chicago, Illinois, in 1891. He married Grace Crampton (1877–1968) in Oregon, Holt County, Missouri, in 1896 and opened a medical practice in Kahoka, Clark County, Missouri. He became secretary of the Northeast Missouri Medical Association in 1897, performed postgraduate work at Rush Medical College during the summer of 1899, and joined the faculty of Keokuk Medical College in 1905 as a professor of physiology and histology. In 1909, Republican Governor Herbert S. Hadley (1872–1927) appointed him to the Missouri State

Board of Health, where his peers elected him their secretary for the next four years (1909–1913). He then moved to Kansas City and practiced medicine there until his death in 1934 at the age of sixty-five years. He was an active member of both the Grand Lodge of the Knights of Pythias in the Grand Domain of Missouri and the Republican Party. He had no children. See Board of the Health of the State of Missouri, Missouri, *Annual Report of the Board of Health of the State of Missouri for 1891* (Jefferson City, MO: Tribune Printing Company, 1892), 45; and "Rush Medical College," *Medical Standard* 22 (1899): 631.

37. Hospital and Health Board, *Second Annual Report of the Board of Hospital and Health of Kansas City, Missouri, for Fiscal Year April 20, 1909, to April 19, 1910, Inclusive* (Kansas City, MO: Kansas City Board of Hospital and Health, 1910), 101.

38. Of note, in April and May 1910, the Kansas City newspapers reported that meningitis was one among several possible causes under consideration in the death of Colonel Thomas Swope during the murder trial of Dr. Bennet Clark Hyde, the Swope family physician and the husband of one of Mr. Swope's nieces. Meningitis was never proved to be the cause of his death. See "Walsh Questions Hektoen; The Afternoon Session Brought a Brisk Cross-Examination," *Kansas City Star*, April 30, 1910, 1; "Defense Expert On; Convulsions in Typhoid; Swope's Ailments Grave," *Kansas City Star*, May 5, 1910, 1.

39. Of note, Dr. Frank Hall declared on October 30, 1911, that "serum as a cure for spinal meningitis" had been used by Kansas City physicians for "nearly two years," thereby suggesting that the serum's first use in Kansas City occurred in October or November of 1909. The authors have been unable to find materials to validate Dr. Hall's claim. See "Meningitis Serum Used Here; Dr. Frank Hall Says the Flexner Treatment Is Not New Here," *Kansas City Star*, October 30, 1911, 5.

40. "Internes," Hospital and Health Board, *Second Annual Report of the Board of Hospital and Health of Kansas City, Missouri, for Fiscal Year April 20, 1909, to April 19, 1910, Inclusive* (Kansas City, MO: Kansas City Board of Hospital and Health, 1910), 26–27.

41. "A Hospital Head Tuesday; The New Superintendent Must Devote All His Time to His Duties," *Kansas City Star*, July 17, 1910, 4; "Hospital's Head a Veteran," *Kansas City Star*, July 20, 1910, 3.

42. Dr. Louis Willard Luscher (1858–1922) was born in Macon County, Missouri, as the third of the four sons of John Henry Luscher (1825–1912), a farmer, and Emily C. Torrey (1831–1900). Louis Luscher attended public schools; earned his bachelor's degree from the Kansas State University in Lawrence, Douglas County, Kansas; and earned his medical diploma from the Kansas City Medical College in 1879 at the age of twenty-one years. He joined the United States Army and served as a surgeon during Native American uprisings on the plains of the United States. He went abroad and served as the chief surgeon of the Chinese government (Army of Formosa) during the Franco-Chinese War (1884–1885). After these and other colorful international exploits, he practiced general medicine for more than two decades in Kansas City, Jackson County, Missouri; served on the medical staff of three Kansas City hospitals; and served as the superintendent of the Kansas City General Hospital (1910–1912). Four years before his death, he retired from medical practice to become treasurer of the Country Club Laundry. He married Charlotte D. Hall (1871–1958) in 1892; they had no children. Dr. Luscher died of a cerebral hemorrhage at home at the age of sixty-four years. See "Luscher, Louis Willard," in Howard Louis Conard, ed., *Encyclopedia of the History of Missouri: A Compendium of History* (New York: Southern History Company, 1901), 4:135–36; "Death of Dr. L. W. Luscher," *Kansas City Star*, December 26, 1922, 2; "Kansas City General Hospital," *Medical Herald* 31, no. 10 (October 1912): 533–34; "Under a Cloak of Religion; Another Side to the Boxer Troubles in China; Dr. L. W. Luscher, Who Spent Several Years in China, Says Many Outlaws Become the Wards of Missionaries Purely to Evade the Law," *Kansas City Star*, June 29, 1900, 12.

43. "Died When a Cure Was Near; A Shipment of Antitoxin Didn't Arrive in Time to Save Two Children," *Kansas City Star*, February 13, 1911, 1.

44. St. Louis City Hospital physicians first used Flexner antimeningitis serum in January 1908 to treat a parturient woman who presented to the hospital with far-advanced symptoms of cerebrospinal meningitis. The hospital physicians telegraphed Dr. Flexner in New York City, who sent vials of antimeningitis serum to St. Louis forthwith. The woman gave birth to a four-pound daughter around January 26, 1908. Despite the use of Flexner antimeningitis serum, the woman died on February 5, 1908. Her daughter died of

THE KANSAS CITY MENINGITIS EPIDEMIC, 1911-1913:

malnutrition at the age of nineteen days. See "Flexner Serum Fails to Save Life of Woman; Mrs. Ellison Succumbs in City Hospital to Spinal Meningitis; Her Baby Is Isolated; Physicians and Nurses Think Thriving Child Has Passed Danger," *St. Louis Post-Dispatch*, February 5, 1908, 4; "Doctors Fight Hard for Baby's Life; Mother Dies; Father Paces Hospital Ward a Widower, Praying for the Child While the Surgeons Work Heroically," *St. Louis-Dispatch*, February 9, 1908, 22; "Baby Winning Fight with Spinal Meningitis, Which Killed Mother in Hospital," *St. Louis Post-Dispatch*, February 10, 1908, 3; and "Starvation Kills Baby as It Conquers Spinal Meningitis; Mrs. Ellison's Daughter, Born as Mother Dies in Hospital, Succumbs to Malnutrition," St. *Louis Post-Dispatch*, February 12, 1908, 3.

45. St. Joseph (St. Joseph's) Hospital opened in 1874 as the first private hospital in Kansas City. Dr. Jefferson Davis Griffith (1850–1924) originated the idea for the hospital. He was born in Jackson, Hinds County, Mississippi, as the eldest of the four children of Sallie Anne Eliza Whitfield (1825–1902) and Richard Griffith (1814–1862), a banker and an adjutant on the staff of President Jefferson Davis of the Confederate States of America. Brigadier General Richard Griffith died at the age of forty-eight years while leading the Seventh Mississippi Brigade in Richmond, Wise County, Virginia, during the American Civil War. Young Jefferson Davis Griffith received his early formal education at the Summerville (Mississippi) Institute, a boys' school established in 1857 ten miles from Macon, Noxubee County, Mississippi. He then enrolled in the Medical Department of the University of the City of New York, where he earned his medical degree in 1871. He served an internship at the Bellevue Hospital (1871–1872) before moving to Kansas City to practice medicine. Seeing only the tiny city hospital in existence there (the original Kansas City Municipal Hospital) at Twenty-Second and McCoy Streets, Dr. Griffith (not a Catholic himself) approached Reverend Father Bernard Donnelly, the pastor of the Church of the Immaculate Conception (on Broadway between Eleventh and Twelfth Streets), about inviting the Sisters of St. Joseph of Carondelet (St. Louis, Missouri) to open a hospital in the old Waterman home, a ten-room residence at Seventh and Pennsylvania Streets in the Quality Hill neighborhood of Kansas City. Father Donnelly (1810–1880) was born in Kilnacreevy, County Cavan, Ireland, as a son of John Donnelly and Rose Fox; he immigrated to the United States from Liverpool, England, in 1842 at the age of thirty-two years and made his way to

Kansas City in the 1850s. He was ordained in St. Louis, Missouri, in 1845. Upon Dr. Griffith's request, Father Donnelly soon welcomed Mother Celestia and three Sisters of St. Joseph of Carondelet to Kansas City, where they opened the hospital with twenty beds and soon added additions to the hospital to increase its capacity to 150 beds. In 1917, the sisters and physicians departed Quality Hill to open a new 250-bed St. Joseph Hospital on Linwood Boulevard and Prospect Street. Both Dr. Griffith and Reverend Donnelly died at their beloved St. Joseph Hospital at the ages of seventy-four and seventy years, respectively. See "Jefferson Davis Griffith, MD," in Walter Barlow Stevens, *Centennial History of Missouri, The Center State, 1821–1915* (Chicago, IL: S. J. Clarke Publishing Company, 1915) 4:249–50; "Jefferson Davis Griffith," in Arthur Wayne Hafner, *Directory of Deceased American Physicians, 1804–1929* (Chicago, IL: American Medical Association, c. 1993); William J. Dalton, *Life of Father Bernard Donnelly with Historical Sketches of Kansas City, St. Louis, and Independence, Missouri* (Kansas City, MO: Grimes-Joyce Printing Company, 1921); Carrie Westlake Whitney, *Kansas City Missouri, Its History and Its People, 1800–1908* (Chicago, IL: S. J. Clarke Publishing Company, 1908), 1:52, 149, 403–7, 478; "The Education and Care of the 'Dear Neighbor' for 145 Years in KC," *Catholic Key Online News 2018*, accessed May 20, 2018, http://catholickey.org/2011/03/31/the-education-and-care-of-the-%E2%80%9Cdear-neighbor%E2%80%9D-for-145-years-in-kc/; and Marion Lott, "CSJ History in KC: Celebrating 150 Years in Kansas City," Sisters of St. Joseph of Carondelet, St. Louis Province, Missouri, accessed May 20, 2018, http://www.csjsl.org/ways-to-act/in-ministry/celebrate-kansas-city-150-years/csj-history-in-kc.php.

46. "The Shannons Won Easily," *Kansas City Times*, March 22, 1911, 10.

47. "JAP Barbeau's Son Is Dead; Spinal Meningitis Brought an End to Third Baseman's Child Last Night," *Kansas City Times*, April 3, 1911, 10.

48. "A Victory Over Meningitis; The Serum Treatment Cures a Man at the General Hospital," *Kansas City Star*, April 9, 1911, 3.

49. Hospital and Health Board, "Medical Diseases—General Hospital," *Third Annual Report of the Hospital and Health Board for Fiscal Year April 18, 1910, to April 17, 1911, Inclusive* (Kansas City, MO: Hospital and Health Board, 1911), 117, 120.

50. The prevalence of cerebrospinal meningitis disease in Kansas City for the winter and spring of 1910–1911 calculates to 0.2 afflicted residents per 10,000 residents, using the total population of the city as 300,000 people.

51. "More Victories Over Death; A Serum Reduces the Proportion of Fatal Meningitis," *Kansas City Star*, May 4, 1911, 3.

52. "New Serum Successful; Antimeningitis Remedy Has Been Generally Accepted by Authorities," *Evening Missourian* (Columbia, MO), May 22, 1911, 2; and Thomas Lynch, "Cerebrospinal Meningitis— Treatment," *Medical Herald* 31, no. 6 (June 1912): 296–98.

53. Dr. Abraham Sophian (1885–1957) was born in Kiev, Russia, as the fifth of the six children of Morris Sophian (1849–1910), a commercial hauler, and Mathilda "Tillie" Pargomeschuk (or Pergamisherig) (1855–1920). Abraham immigrated at the age of five years to New York City with his family, grew up in an apartment in a five-story redbrick building at 265 Henry Street, attended nearby public schools on the Lower East Side of Manhattan, completed the five-year combined secondary-collegiate program at the College of the City of New York in 1902 at the age of seventeen years, won a competitive state scholarship to attend Cornell University Medical College in New York City for four years, and graduated from Cornell University Medical College in 1906 at the age of twenty-one years. He subsequently won by competitive examination a place on the medical house staff of New York City's Mount Sinai Hospital, serving there from January 1, 1907, to June 30, 1909. He next won a George Blumenthal Jr. Fellowship, which he served in the pathology department of Mount Sinai Hospital in New York City from July 1, 1909, to June 30, 1910. He then joined the Research Laboratory of the New York City Board of Health as the head of its meningitis division on July 1, 1910. He wed Estelle Felix (1882– 1970) on Wednesday, April 26, 1911. On Wednesday, January 3, 1912, he boarded a train to Dallas, Dallas County, Texas, where he assisted in the control of the cerebrospinal meningitis epidemic underway there. See "Visiting Doctors Hear Dr. Sophian; Many from Other Texas Cities Attend Dinner by Physicians' Lunch Club; Treatment of Disease; Advises Administering Meningitis Serum on First Day—Outlines Precautions Advisable," *Dallas Morning News*, January 7, 1912, 8.

54. Phebe L. DuBois, "Differential Diagnosis and Treatment of Epidemic Cerebrospinal Meningitis," *Journal of the American Medical Association* 60, no. 11 (March 15, 1913): 820–22.

55. Henry Kendall Mulford (1866–1937) was born in Bridgeton, Cumberland County, New Jersey, as the eldest of the three sons of Joseph Lewis Mulford (1844–1912), a tinsmith, and Adeline Brooks Nieukirk (1846–1893). He graduated from the South Jersey Institute in 1884 and from the Philadelphia College of Pharmacy, the first pharmacy school in North America (founded in 1821), in 1887. He purchased a small drugstore, founded the H. K. Mulford Company, and became the first commercial entity in the United States to manufacture antitoxins and vaccines. After retiring, he founded the Mulford Colloid Laboratory, and he remained its president until his death. He also was a director of the Research and Biological Laboratories of the National Drug Company. He married Lillian Bell Ware (1866–1945) in 1890; they had three children. He died of heart disease at the age of seventy-one years. "Henry Kendall Mulford," *Pennsylvania Medical Journal* 41, no. 2 (November 1937): 174; and "H. K. Mulford Dies; Pharmacy Pioneer: Company He Founded Was First to Make Anti-Toxins," *Philadelphia Inquirer*, October 16, 1937, 4.

56. See Louis Galambos, *Networks of Innovation: Vaccine Development at Merck, Sharp and Dohme, and Mulford, 1895–1995* (New York: Cambridge University Press, 1997).

57. See H. K. Mulford, "The Preparation of Diphtheria Antitoxic Serum," *Proceedings of the American Pharmaceutical Association at the Forty-Fourth Annual Meeting Held at Montreal, Canada, August 1896* (Baltimore, MD: American Pharmaceutical Association, 1896): 227–31.

58. Jonathan Liebenau, "Selling Science: The H. K. Mulford Company," *Medical Science and Medical Industry: Studies in Business History* (London: Palgrave Macmillan, 1987), 57–58.

59. "Minutes, State Board of Health, Jefferson City, Mo., July 14, 1911," State Board of Health of Missouri, *Twenty-Ninth Annual Report of the State Board of Health of Missouri 1911* (Jefferson City, MO: Hugh Stephens Printing Company, 1911), 36.

60. Dr. Ernest Franklin Robinson (1872–1945) was born in Lawrence, Douglas County, Kansas, as the eldest of the four children of David Hamilton Robinson (1837–1895), the first professor of Greek and Latin at the University of Kansas (Lawrence, Douglas County,

Kansas), and Henrietta Beach (1849–1906). Ernest Robinson earned his bachelor's degree from the University of Kansas and his medical degree from the University of Pennsylvania School of Medicine in 1896. He opened a medical practice in Philadelphia and served an extended term at the City Hospital and at St. Agnes Hospital, both also in Philadelphia. He subsequently became the surgeon for the Burlington Railroad, the chief surgeon for the Kansas City Terminal Railway Company (1903–1915), and the president of the Missouri State Board of Health (1909–1914). He married Mary Burnet Kip (1876–1923) in 1904; they had three children. "Dr. Ernest Franklin Robinson, Kansas Alpha, 1888," *Shield of Phil Kappa Psi* (November 1944): 160; *Olathe Mirror* (Olathe, KS), August 11, 1898, 2; "Dr. Ernest F. Robinson Dies," *Moberly Monitor-Index* (Moberly, MO), February 6, 1945, 7; and "Former State Board of Health President Dies," *Macon Chronicle-Herald* (Macon, MO), February 6, 1945, 6.

61. Dr. Milton Pleam Overholser (1859–1937) was born in Will County, Illinois, as one of the six children of Levi Overholser (1833–1923) and Maria C. Pleam (1832–1893). His place of medical training is not known at the present time. He was a member of the State Board of Health of Missouri (1909–1911); superintendent of the State Hospital for the Insane (No. 3) in Nevada, Missouri (1911–1913); and superintendent of the State Hospital at St. Joseph (1927–1930). He married Fannie E. Long (1866–1919) in 1887; they had two children. He subsequently married Leila Britt (1869–1944). He died of prostate cancer at the age of seventy-eight years. "Prominent Doctor Dies," *Moberly Monitor-Index* (Moberly, MO), June 19, 1937, 4.

62. Dr. Louis Edward Bunte (1872–1964) was born in Rosebud, Gasconade County, Missouri, as one of the six children of Herman E. Bunte (1841–1908), a farmer, and Elise Mellies (1841–1911). He was a prominent homeopathist, secretary of the St. Louis Homeopathic Medical Society, a member of the Missouri Institute of Homeopathy, and a member of the State Board of Health of Missouri (1909–1913). He practiced medicine in St. Louis until 1937, when he moved his practice to Marshall, Saline County, Missouri. He retired in 1952 and died in 1964 at the age of ninety-two years. "Services to Be Saturday for Dr. Louis E. Bunte," *St. Louis Post-Dispatch*, June 11, 1964, 26; and "Missouri," *Journal of the American Institute of Homoeopathy* 1, no. 9 (September 1909): 444.

63. The authors could find no further discussion of the Mulford proposal in subsequent minutes of the board.

64. "Four New Meningitis Cases," *Kansas City Star*, March 7, 1912, 6.

65. "Minutes, State Board of Health, Jefferson City, Mo., July 14, 1911," State Board of Health of Missouri, *Twenty-Ninth Annual Report of the State Board of Health of Missouri 1911* (Jefferson City, MO: Hugh Stephens Printing Company, 1911), 36–37.

66. In 1911, Dr. Luscher wrote, "I have to thank my processor for his selection of a class of bright and well-equipped young men as interns, by competitive examination. Graduates in medicine from many of the best colleges in America, who, one and all, have entered heartily into their work in diagnosing diseases and assuming personal care of the sick. Their work cannot be too highly commended. The plan of selection has proven so advantageous that I have, this year adopted the same method, and hope to be able to secure the services of a group of men equally serviceable." Hospital and Health Board, *Third Annual Report of the Hospital and Health Board of Kansas City, Missouri, for Fiscal Year April 18, 1910, to April 17, 1911, Inclusive* (Kansas City, MO: Hospital and Health Board, 1911), 95.

67. Dr. Arthur Hawley Parmelee (1883–1961) was born in Redfield, Spink County, South Dakota, as one of the seven children of Joseph Elliot Parmelee (1844–1911), a postmaster, and Martha Elizabeth Dudley (1851–1928). Arthur Parmelee graduated from West Salem High School (West Salem, La Crosse County, Wisconsin) in 1900; worked as a rural mail carrier (1900–1901); played football for and earned his bachelor's degree from Beloit College in Beloit, Rock County, Wisconsin (1905); served as a football coach and secretary of the Young Men's Christian Association at Miami University in Ohio (1906–1907); earned his medical degree from Rush Medical College, which, at the time, was affiliated with the University of Chicago (1911); and served a one-year internship at the Kansas City General Hospital (1911–1912). He joined the practice of Dr. John Cross, an internist, in Minneapolis, Hennepin County, Minnesota, and then moved to Oak Park, Cook County, Illinois, where he practiced general medicine for five years before specializing in pediatrics. He was a member of the medical staff at Children's Memorial Hospital in Chicago (1915–1920) and later served as the chief of pediatrics at both St. Luke's Hospital and Cook County General Hospital in Chicago. He moved to Los Angeles, California, in 1947, where he worked as a full-time pediatrician at Children's Hospital Los

Angeles. He married Ruth Frances Brown (1889–1970) in St. Louis in 1912; they had three children. He died of a cerebral hemorrhage at the age of seventy-eight years. See Philip Rothman, "Arthur Hawley Parmelee, MD, 1883–1961, Pioneer Pediatrician to the Newborn," *American Journal of the Diseases of Children* 103, no. 2 (1962): 197–200; "Dr. Parmelee Taken by Death," *Los Angeles Times*, June 8, 1961, 45; and "The Family Parmelee," accessed October 2, 2017, http://www.thefamilyparmelee.com/x05-1093f.html.

68. Dr. Harry Johnson Schott (1887–1942) was born in Vermillion, Clay County, South Dakota, as the middle of the three sons of Dr. George Schott (1858–1926) and Mary Cynthia (Mamie) Johnson (1861–1946). Harry moved with his family to Sioux City, Woodbury County, Iowa, the year of his birth. He graduated from Sioux City High School and earned his bachelor of science degree from the University of Chicago in 1907, where he played football under the famous coach Amos Alonzo Stagg (1862–1965). He earned his medical degree from Rush Medical College, which, at the time, was associated with the University of Chicago, in 1909; served an internship at the Kansas City General Hospital (1911–1912); and moved back to Sioux City to practice orthopedic surgery. In 1915, he gave a speech titled "Observations on Epidemic Cerebrospinal Meningitis" at the Twentieth Annual Session of the Sioux Valley Medical Association in Sioux Valley, South Dakota [*sic*]. The speech does not survive. He moved to Los Angeles in 1921 to join the medical staff of the Orthopaedic Hospital and St. Vincent's Hospital. He married Helen Josephine Holman (1888–1972) in 1912; they had one child. Dr. Schott died at the age of fifty-five years at St. Vincent's Hospital after a year's illness. See "Doctors of the Sioux Valley to Meet Here; Twentieth Annual Convention to Open Tomorrow for Two Days' Session," *Argus-Leader* (Sioux Falls, SD), July 20, 1915; and "Dr. H. J. Schott Called by Death; Chief Orthopaedic Consultant of City Schools Succumbs," *Los Angeles Times*, November 25, 1942, 8.

69. Dr. Frederick Worley Aves (1886–1962) was born in Norwalk, Huron County, Ohio, as the middle child of the five children of Reverend Charles S. Aves (1851–1923), an Episcopal minister, and Jessie Olivia Hughes (1863–1935). In 1902, the family moved to Texas, where Reverend Aves became rector of Trinity Episcopal Church in Galveston and helped to rebuild the church after the Galveston hurricane of 1900. Fred W. Aves studied at Kenyon College

in Gambier, Knox County, Ohio, and earned his medical degree from the University of Texas Medical Branch at Galveston in 1911. He won an internship to the Kansas City General Hospital (1911–1912) by competitive examination. The next year, he worked at Kensington Hospital for Women in Philadelphia, Pennsylvania, and studied for three months (postgraduate training) at the University of Pennsylvania. In 1913, he returned to Galveston to become an instructor in surgery at the University of Texas Medical Branch. Six years later, in 1919, he resigned this post and devoted his time to his private practice. He married Florence Louise Huston (1888–1988) in 1913; they had three children. Dr. Aves died of a ruptured abdominal aneurysm at the age of seventy-six years. See "Dr. F. W. Aves," in Ellis Arthur Davis and Edwin H. Grobe, *New Encyclopedia of Texas* (Dallas, TX: Texas Development Bureau, 1926), 2:1375.

70. Dr. Frank Randall Teachenor (1888–1953) was born in Kansas City, Jackson County, Missouri, as one of the two sons of Richard Bennington Teachenor (1864–1942), an engraver, and Mary Catherine Givaudin (1867–1947). He entered the University of Kansas School of Medicine directly from high school; earned his medical degree in 1911; served an internship (1911–1912) at the Kansas City General Hospital; and joined the practice of Dr. Jabez Jackson, a Kansas City surgeon. He served in France during World War I after obtaining training in neurosurgery at the University of Pennsylvania. After returning to the United States, he provided neurosurgical care for all of the hospitals in the Kansas City area as well as much of the Midwest. He was the first chief of neurosurgery at the University of Kansas Medical Center, serving from 1921 to 1951. He married Ethel G. Heath (1889–1949) in 1920; they had one child. Dr. Teachenor died from a heart attack on his way to work; he was sixty-five years old. See Charles E. Brackett, "Frank Teachenor, MD, Pioneer Neurosurgeon," Medicine in the First World War, KU Medical Center, University of Kansas, accessed February 9, 2018, http://www.kumc.edu/wwi/essays-on-first-world-war-medicine/index-of-essays/biography/frank-teachnor.html.

71. Dr. Benjamin Weems Turner (1889–1972) was born in Bonney, Brazoria County, Texas, as one of the three children of Francis Williamson Turner (1856–1943), a stockman, and Annie Dorothy Krause (1863–1944). He earned his medical degree from the University of Texas Medical Branch at Galveston (1991), served his internship at the Kansas City General Hospital (1911–1912),

and served a residency in urological surgery at the Johns Hopkins University Hospital in Baltimore, Maryland, under the guidance of Dr. Hugh Hampton Young (1870–1945). Dr. Turner opened a urological practice in Houston, Texas, in 1913 and established the Turner Urological Institute, a twenty-two-bed hospital modeled after the Brady Urological Institute at Johns Hopkins University School of Medicine (established in 1915). Dr. Turner married Margaret Carnes in 1915; they had three children. He died at the age of eighty-three years. See William D. Steers, "Turner, Benjamin Weems," *Handbook of Texas Online*, accessed February 9, 2018, https://tshaonline.org/handbook/online/articles/ftu15.

72. Dr. Richard Williams Spicer Sr. (1887–1960) was born in Goldsboro, Wayne County, North Carolina, as one of the dozen children of Dr. John Daniel Spicer (1840–1908) and Emma Fedora Williams (1840–1919). Richard Spicer earned his bachelor's degree from Davidson College in Davidson, Mecklenburg County, North Carolina, and his medical degree from the University of Pennsylvania in Philadelphia (1911). He served two years on the house staff of the Kansas City General Hospital (1911–1913); practiced medicine in Hazelton, Luzerne County, Pennsylvania; and moved back to Goldsboro, North Carolina, to join his brothers in their medical practice. He married Stuart Hayden Rogers (1896–1987) in 1931; they had one child. Dr. Spicer died of heart disease at the age of seventy-two years. See "Dr. Spicer, Winston-Salem, Weds Mrs. Stuart Rogers," *Greensboro Daily News* (Greensboro, NC), September 1, 1931, 8; and W. J. Maxwell, *General Alumni Catalogue of the University of Pennsylvania, 1917* (Philadelphia, PA: Alumni Association of the University, 1917), 856.

73. Dr. Elmer Vail Eyman (1885–1955) was born in Madison, Dane County, Wisconsin, as one of the two sons of Franklin Pierce Eyman (1854–1931), a railroad agent, and Alice Thurza Prickett (1858–1920). He earned his bachelor's degree at the University of Wisconsin in 1907 and his medical degree from Rush Medical College in 1911. He was associated with the Pennsylvania Hospital in Philadelphia (1919–1950) and served as the chief of services of the hospital's department for mental and nervous diseases for twenty years. He pioneered the development of the Pennsylvania Hospital School of Nursing for Men, which graduated 550 men during its fifty-one-year history. Dr. Eyman married Euretta Sophia Sheldon (1890–1982) in 1920; they had two children. He died of heart disease at the age of

seventy years. *University of Wisconsin Alumni Directory, 1849–1911* (Madison, WI: University of Wisconsin, 1912), 122; "Dr. Elmer V. Eyman," *Courier-Post* (Camden, NJ), February 14, 1955, 4; "Dr. E. V. Eyman Dies on His Birthday," *Philadelphia Inquirer,* February 14, 1955, 6; and "School of Nursing for Men, Class of 1924," Penn Medicine, History of Pennsylvania Hospital, accessed February 9, 2018, http://www.uphs.upenn.edu/paharc/collections/gallery/people/Male_Students.html.

74. Dr. Franklin E. Murphy (1867–1933) was born in Indiana as the eldest of the four children of Dr. Hugh C. Murphy (1843–1903) and Martha J. Cook (1844–1935). The family moved to Missouri when Franklin Murphy was young. He earned his medical degree from the University of Pennsylvania School of Medicine in 1893; moved to Kansas City; opened a medical practice; and became a founding member of the medical faculty of the University of Kansas School of Medicine in Rosedale, Wyandotte County, Kansas, in 1910. He was a professor of internal medicine at the university and served as an attending physician at the Kansas City General Hospital, a president of Jackson County Medical Society, and a member of the Missouri State Board of Health. He married Cordelia Brown (1880–1947) in 1915; they had three children. He died at the age of sixty-six years. See "Dr. Franklin E. Murphy Dies," *St. Louis Post-Dispatch*, February 21, 1933, 17; "End Comes to Instructor in KU Medical School," *Hutchinson News* (Hutchinson, KS), February 21, 1933, 6; W. J. Maxwell, *General Alumni Catalogue of the University of Pennsylvania* (Philadelphia, PA: Alumni Association of the University, 1917), 769; and "Hyde's Wealth of Symptoms," *Kansas City Star*, April 24, 1910, 8.

75. Dr. Hugh D. Hamilton (1872–1926) was born in Crab Orchard, Ray County, Missouri, as one of the four children of Thomas Hamilton (1824–1886), a farmer, and Sarah Clark (1835–1933). Hugh D. Hamilton attended the Woodson Institute in Richmond, Ray County, Missouri, and earned his medical diploma in 1898 after attending the Missouri Medical College and the McDowell Medical College in St. Louis, Missouri. He married Bertha W. McCrosky (1876–1958) in 1902; they had two children. Dr. Hamilton died of renal cancer at the age of fifty-five years in St. Joseph Hospital, Kansas City. He was part owner of the Frick Ice Cream Company in Corsicana, Texas. See "Arthur W. Hafner," in Arthur Wayne Hafner, *Directory of*

Deceased American Physicians, 1804–1929 (Chicago, IL: American Medical Association, c. 1993).

76. Dr. John Lincoln Robinson (1861–1936) was born in either Iowa or Kansas as one of the half dozen children of Levi Robinson (1839–1895), a farmer, and Mary F. Bradley (1841–1898). John Lincoln Robinson earned his medical diploma from the University Medical College of Kansas City in 1884 and studied at the College of Physicians and Surgeons of New York City for at least one year (1887–1888). He married Annie Elizabeth Sote (1867–1942); they had no children. He practiced medicine for fifty years in Kansas City and died at the age of seventy-five years at the Research Hospital in Kansas City after a short illness. See *Annual Catalogue and Announcement of College of Physicians and Surgeons in the City of New York, Medical Department of Columbia College* (New York: Macgowan and Slipper, 1888), 15; and "Dr. John L. Robinson Dies at Kansas City," *Sedalia Weekly Democrat*, October 16, 1936, 5.

77. Dr. Frederick McKendrie Lowe (1871–1937) was born in Lathrop, Clinton County, Missouri, as the youngest of the three children of William McKendrie Lowe (1833–1923), a farmer, and Harriet Ellen Lowe (1834–1912). Frederick Lowe attended the State Normal School of Missouri in Warrensburg, Johnson County, Missouri, for two years (1893–1895) and Harvard College for two years (1893–1895), earning his bachelor of science degree at the latter in 1895. He taught chemistry and physics at the Shattuck Military Academy in Faribault, Rice County, Minnesota, for five years before attending Rush Medical College, which, at the time, was associated with the University of Chicago, where he earned his medical degree in 1903. He served an internship at the Milwaukee Hospital in Milwaukee, Milwaukee County, Wisconsin; opened a medical practice in Brownwood, Brown County, Texas; taught chemistry at Howard Payne College in Brownwood, Texas; moved to Kansas City to open a medical practice in 1907; and began caring for patients at the Kansas City General Hospital in 1908. He married Mary Myrtle Osborne, the head of the English department at the Missouri State Normal School, in 1906; they had no children. Failing vision in 1925 forced his retirement. He died in 1937 at the age of sixty-six years. See "Frederick McKendrie Lowe," *Harvard College Class of 1895 Fifth Report* (Cambridge, MA: Crimson, 1915), 188; and "Frederick McKendrie Lowe," *Harvard College Class of 1895, Thirty-Fifth*

Anniversary Report (Cambridge, MA: Tolman-University Press, 1930), 62.

78. Dr. Charles Clinton Conover (1871–1962) was born in Peculiar, Cass County, Missouri, as one of the seven children of Dr. Richard Ashton Conover (1831–1886), a Civil War general, and Sarah Fisher (1833–1924), a trained nurse. He earned his bachelor's degree in agriculture at the University of Missouri in 1896. While in college, he established football records as a halfback and as one of the finest breakaway runners in Missouri football history. He then served as a high school principal for two years in Shelbina, Shelby County, Missouri, before moving to Kansas City in 1899 to attend the University Medical College of Kansas City, where he earned his medical diploma in 1901. He next served as the house surgeon of Kansas City Municipal Hospital (1901–1905); studied with Dr. Richard Cabot (1868–1939) at the Massachusetts General Hospital in Boston; and returned to Kansas City to practice medicine for the next fifty years. He taught at the University of Kansas Medical School and served on the medical staff of Trinity Lutheran Hospital for thirty years. He married Perla Mae Petty (1879–1970) in 1903; they had two children. He developed a strong interest in psychosomatic medicine. See "Dr. Charles Conover; Doctor Here More than 50 Years Was 90; Laboratory at Trinity Lutheran Hospital Named after Him," *Kansas City Times*, August 24, 1961, 3.

79. Dr. Scott Parker Child (1867–1940) was born in Littleton, Grafton Count, New Hampshire, as one of the seven children of Parker Morse Child (1838–1926), a life insurance agent, and Abigail Hatch (born in 1841). The family moved to Neponset, Bureau County, Illinois, when Scott Child was young. He attended Oberlin College Preparatory School (1887–1888) in Oberlin, Loraine County, Ohio; Oberlin College (1888–1892, 1897), from which he earned a bachelor of philosophy degree (1892) and a master's degree (1897); and the University of Pennsylvania School of Medicine, from which he earned his medical degree in 1896. He moved to Kansas City, opened a medical practice, and married Mary Townsend Hotchkiss in 1901; they had no children. He died at the age of seventy-three years. See "Scott P. Child," in W. J. Maxwell, *General Alumni Catalogue of the University of Pennsylvania* (Philadelphia, PA: Alumni Association of the University, 1917), 784.

80. Hospital and Health Board, *Fourth Annual Report of the Hospital and Health Board of Kansas City, Missouri, for Fiscal Year April*

17, 1911, to April 15, 1912, Inclusive (Kansas City, MO: Hospital and Health Board, 1912), 5.

81. "Every Disease to Itself; Conveniences in the New Contagion Hospital; Two Buildings Will Be Connected by a 1-Story Receiving Department with Sun Porches on Top—Construction to Start This Week," *Kansas City Star*, August 13, 1911, 3.

82. "A Smallpox Victim Complains; City's Contagious Hospital Sent a Woman to Negro Institution," *Kansas City Star*, March 28, 1913, 4.

83. "Contagion Hospital Ready January 1," *Kansas City Star*, December 18, 1912, 2.

84. "Meningitis Serum Used Here; Dr. Frank Hall Says the Flexner Treatment Is Not New Here," *Kansas City Star*, October 30, 1911, 5.

CHAPTER 2

THE COZY, FOX, AND SWAN
ROOMING HOUSES, JANUARY 1912

The winter of 1912 in Kansas City was one of the coldest and snowiest in the city's recorded history.[1] City residents mostly remained indoors, often in unventilated buildings, and a large number of the rural poor moved into Kansas City to obtain food and shelter. Kansas City's health commissioner, Dr. Wheeler, bemoaned the transient poor for spending the winter inside of cheap, unsanitary, crowded tenements and lodging houses, which he identified as the breeding grounds for contagious diseases.[2-3]

On Friday, January 5, 1912, five-year-old Cynthia Marvin Green, the only child of a bookkeeper and his wife, succumbed to cerebrospinal meningitis at home after a short illness.[4] Her death by itself probably would have passed unnoticed if not for the *Kansas City Star*'s breaking story three days later on Monday, January 8, 1912, about the raging Texas cerebrospinal meningitis epidemic in Waco, Texas, 540 miles (as the crow flies) southwest of Kansas City.[5] Fifty-five people in Waco had died from the disease since Friday, December 15, 1911. Kansas City maintained strong commercial ties with the cities of Texas and other southwestern states. A constant stream of people and goods traveled the railroads between Kansas City and these other cities. Dr. Wheeler realized the cerebrospinal meningitis epidemic in Waco threatened Kansas City.[6]

On Saturday, January 13, 1912, Dr. Luscher admitted a person with possible cerebrospinal meningitis to the Kansas City General Hospital. Yet the situation was confusing. Since Friday, December 1, 1911, Dr. Luscher believed that hospital physicians actually had treated seven or eight people with meningitis while incorrectly calling their illnesses pneumonia. Three of the patients had died. Only one of three dead patients had proven cerebrospinal meningitis, according to the death certificate, meaning that a physician had obtained a cerebrospinal fluid sample, either before death via a lumbar puncture procedure or after death during autopsy, to establish the diagnosis as cerebrospinal meningitis.[7]

When Dr. Wheeler learned about the admission of the patient with cerebrospinal meningitis to Kansas City General Hospital on Saturday, January 13, 1912, and about the possibility of seven or eight cases of the disease occurring between Friday, December 1, 1911, and January 13, 1911, as detected by Dr. Luscher, he asked Dr. William Lucien Gist,[8] one of his assistant administrators, to review the physician diagnoses on Kansas City death certificates possessed by the Hospital and Health Board between Monday, May 1, 1911, and Saturday, December 30, 1911 [sic]. It is likely that Dr. Wheeler chose this time interval for his retrospective review to accord with his department's fiscal year, which extended from mid-April 1910 to mid-April 1911. What did Dr. Gist learn?

Dr. Gist identified the cause of death as simply "meningitis" (i.e., the etiology of the meningitis not specified) on eighteen death certificates during the aforementioned time interval. He could not say whether the meningococcus caused all of the eighteen meningitis deaths; however, using the worst possible scenario, he assumed the meningococcus had caused the eighteen deaths. He then used the mortality rate of 50 percent for cerebrospinal meningitis (his source for using the 50 percent number is not known). He then determined that if eighteen people had died from cerebrospinal meningitis during the aforementioned time interval in 1911, there must have been around thirty-six people with the disease during the aforementioned time interval in 1911.

From this data, the prevalence of cerebrospinal meningitis between May 1, 1911, and December 30, 1911, in Kansas City (using 250,000 as the population of Kansas City) calculated to approximately *1.44 cases of cerebrospinal meningitis per 10,000 Kansas City residents*. This level was not consistent with an epidemic.[9] Furthermore, the 1.44 prevalence was a maximum number, as it is unlikely that the cause of the meningitis was cerebrospinal meningitis in all eighteen individuals who died of their meningitis as noted on the death certificates reviewed by Dr. Gist for the given period.

Dr. Gist and Dr. Wheeler further observed that the eighteen meningitis deaths during the aforementioned time interval in 1911 in Kansas City had been scattered all over the city, a pattern characteristic of cerebrospinal meningitis epidemics.[10] Cerebrospinal meningitis epidemics did not start from a center and radiate in rings outward from that center, as did measles, chickenpox, and smallpox epidemics. This unique behavior of cerebrospinal meningitis epidemics was one of the many reasons why they were difficult to identify and control.

On Saturday, January 20, 1912, as Dr. Luscher, the attending medical staff, and the interns of the Kansas City General Hospital were sorting out the meningitis prevalence situation in their hospital over the previous nine months, Dr. Frank Hall and Dr. Sophian in Kansas City and Dallas, respectively, shared information about the concurrent cerebrospinal meningitis epidemics raging in the two cities.[11] It is unknown who contacted whom or by what means they communicated—telephone, wire, or letter. Recall that Dr. Sophian was the meningitis division director of the Research Laboratory of the New York City Board of Health. With the blessing of the Research Laboratory director Dr. Park and Dr. Flexner of the Rockefeller Institute for Medical Research, he had traveled to Dallas, reaching the city on Friday evening, January 5, 1912, to assist in the control of the cerebrospinal meningitis epidemic there.[12] Soon after his arrival, the mayor of Dallas had ordered the conversion of the sixty-five-bed Dallas City Hospital into a meningitis hospital, where Dr. Sophian, Dr. Albert Ware Nash[13] (the Dallas City health officer), interns, nurses, and orderlies cared for all the afflicted patients they could find in Dallas City and Dallas County.[14]

Dallas's population (92,000 people in 1910[15]) was about one-third the size of the population of Kansas City (about 250,000 people in 1910[16]). The discrepancy in city size notwithstanding, Dr. Hall sought information from Dr. Sophian about his methods of managing the epidemic in Dallas, and Dr. Sophian sought Dr. Hall's opinion on an experimental meningococcal vaccine Dr. Sophian was thinking of manufacturing in Dallas to stem the spread of the epidemic there. The only portion of the two physicians' conversation known to history is their discussion of ways to protect people in constant contact with individuals stricken with cerebrospinal meningitis. Dr. Sophian said that he; many of the physicians, nurses, and orderlies of the Dallas City Hospital; and some of the local Dallas physicians were protecting themselves with a subcutaneous injection of ten cubic centimeters of Flexner antimeningitis serum. No one, said Dr. Sophian, so treated thus far had developed the disease since January 7, 1912, when he first had urged this means of prevention.[17]

Subcutaneous antimeningitis serum had two drawbacks: it was a temporary solution and caused serum sickness (fever, joint pain, and rash)[17] in some people, especially after repeated use. Even though Dr. Sophian himself had developed serum sickness after a subcutaneous injection of Flexner antimeningitis serum, he insisted to Dallas physicians, nurses, and orderlies that "the temporary annoyance of the hives and the very small risk of antiphylaxis [sic] was as nothing compared with the risk and danger of meningitis."[18] What did Dr. Hall think of the subcutaneous injection of Flexner antimeningitis serum to prevent cerebrospinal meningitis? Dr. Hall commended to Dr. Sophian the idea of the subcutaneous injection of Flexner antimeningitis serum to prevent cerebrospinal meningitis in people in constant contact with afflicted individuals.[10]

Dr. Sophian then shared his idea with Dr. Hall of using a heat-killed meningococcal vaccine as a prophylaxis for people in constant contact with afflicted individuals.[19-20] Such a vaccine was not in use at the time in the United States. He stated his belief that a meningococcal vaccine would be safer and longer acting than a subcutaneous injection of Flexner antimeningitis serum and likened such a vaccine to the heat-killed typhoid vaccine originated by Dr. Almroth Edward Wright in 1897 to prevent typhoid fever among British soldiers.[21-23] Dr. Sophian asked Dr. Hall's opinion of a heat-killed meningococcal vaccine as a prophylactic against cerebrospinal meningitis. Dr. Hall commended to Dr. Sophian his idea of a meningococcal vaccine.[10]

Four days passed. On Wednesday, January 24, 1912, Dr. Luscher, eyeing the half-finished contagious-diseases hospital north of the Kansas City General Hospital, converted a third-floor ward in the north building of the hospital into a meningitis ward.[24] This ward contained ten beds in two rows separated by a wide aisle.[25] The interns, attending physicians, nurses, and orderlies working in the meningitis ward wore gowns, masks, head coverings, and gloves[25] to protect against contracting cerebrospinal meningitis. At an unknown time in 1912, Dr. John Roberts VanAtta,[26] the hospital pathologist who had succeeded Dr. Stone, began preparing a heat-killed meningococcal vaccine in the Kansas City General Hospital laboratory to administer to staff members who sought it.[27]

Also, on Wednesday, January 24, 1912, Dr. Luscher publicly acknowledged the admission to the Kansas City General Hospital meningitis ward of eight patients with cerebrospinal meningitis since Monday, January 1, 1912.[24] Three of them were already dead. All current patients in the meningitis ward were receiving Flexner antimeningitis serum. Dr. Luscher also recalled that a decade earlier, all eight patients with cerebrospinal meningitis in the Kansas City Municipal Hospital had died.[28] Now the use of Flexner antimeningitis serum gave patients a chance to survive. He remarked, "If we get the patients in time without any complications, the chances for recovery are pretty good." He added, "This is not exactly an epidemic, but people should be careful, for the unwonted number of cases at present, and the nature of the disease, which is contagious, show that it is a serious problem and precautions should be taken against contracting it."[24]

Dr. Luscher added that most of the people admitted to the Kansas City General Hospital with the disease thus far had come from unsanitary and crowded dwellings and had breathed foul air. "I don't mean to say that such conditions create the germs," he said, "but rather make people more liable to the disease." He warned, "People should stay away from the source of infection, keep their houses clean and sanitary, and above all, breathe pure air."[28]

Cerebrospinal meningitis victims continued to arrive at the Kansas City General Hospital over the next week. On Wednesday, January 24, 1912, Dr. Luscher admitted a thirty-year-old railroad employee named C. H. Sharp, whom Dr. Darwin Delap,[29] a Kansas City ambulance physician, had discovered unconscious in the Fox Hotel at 548 Main Street, Kansas City.[30] Mr. Sharp died within hours of his admission to the Kansas City General Hospital.[31] He was buried in the Leeds Cemetery of Kansas City; his grave was marked with a metal stake, and his name was written on a piece of paper held under a piece of glass.[32]

The next day, Thursday, January 25, 1912, two new victims of cerebrospinal meningitis were admitted to the Kansas City General Hospital.[33] The patients were Curtis E. Greenwood,[34] a twenty-eight-year-old married carpenter, and twenty-year-old Jack Williams, a laborer born in England.[35] Dr. Luscher said that the five patients already in the meningitis ward were doing well, and he hoped "to pull them through."[33] The arrival of these two additional sick men stressed the supply of Flexner antimeningitis serum available to the physicians at the Kansas City General Hospital. Only three entities[36] in the United States produced antimeningitis serum at that time: H. K. Mulford Company, Parke-Davis and Company,[37] and the New York City Board of Health. The wholesale pharmaceutical houses in Kansas City wired for fresh supplies to meet the surging demand.[37]

On Friday, January 26, 1912, the *Public Health Reports*, a weekly periodical published by the United States Public Health

Service[38] in Washington, DC, led with a twenty-five-page primer titled "Epidemic Cerebrospinal Meningitis: A Review of Its Etiology, Transmission, and Specific Therapy, with Reference to Pubic Measures for Its Control."[39] The author was Dr. Wade Hampton Frost,[40] a passed assistant surgeon[41] of the United States Public Health Service.[42] Dr. Frost noted that the cost of antimeningitis serum paled in comparison to the cost of the proper treatment of each case, which required "the daily and almost constant services of at least two physicians and skilled attendants." The most efficient way of providing these services, added Dr. Frost, was to concentrate the patients in a hospital with adequate faciltiies.[43] To prevent the spread of the disease, Dr. Frost advised reporting all cases on suspicion; isolating afflicted patients; disinfecting noses and throats with antiseptics; minimizing communication between the infected and the exposed; closing schools; avoiding large public gatherings; avoiding the use of public drinking cups; and administering urotropin.[44-45]

On Saturday, January 27, 1912, the Hospital and Health Board, having received no reports of new cerebrospinal meningitis cases during the previous thirty-six hours, declared that the meningitis "scare" was over.[46] Dr. Wheeler assured Kansas City residents that the city was taking "every precaution to prevent the spread of the disease" by observing "all cheap rooming houses and hotels" and by fumigating every place where cases had developed. He also informed the general public about the confinement of all meningitis patients in a single meningitis ward of the Kansas City General Hospital and the exercise of caution by attendants in that ward while caring for patients with the disease.[46]

Hours after the Hospital and Health Board announced the end of the meningitis scare on Saturday, January 27, 1912, three new meningitis-afflicted individuals arrived at the Kansas City General Hospital.[47] The first was thirty-eight-year-old James Carroll, a laborer and resident of Cozy House at 24 East Third Street, Kansas City.[47] The second was H. A Davis, a thirty-year-old laborer staying at the Fox Hotel at 548 Main Street, Kansas City.[48] Mr. Davis walked into the Emergency Hospital,[49] which was located in the basement of the nearby City Hall,[50] to seek treatment, whence he was transported post haste to the meningitis ward of the Kansas City General Hospital.[48] The third person with cerebrospinal meningitis was nineteen-year-old Leo Griffin,[51] a railroad worker who lived with his family at 3023 Michigan Avenue, Kansas City.

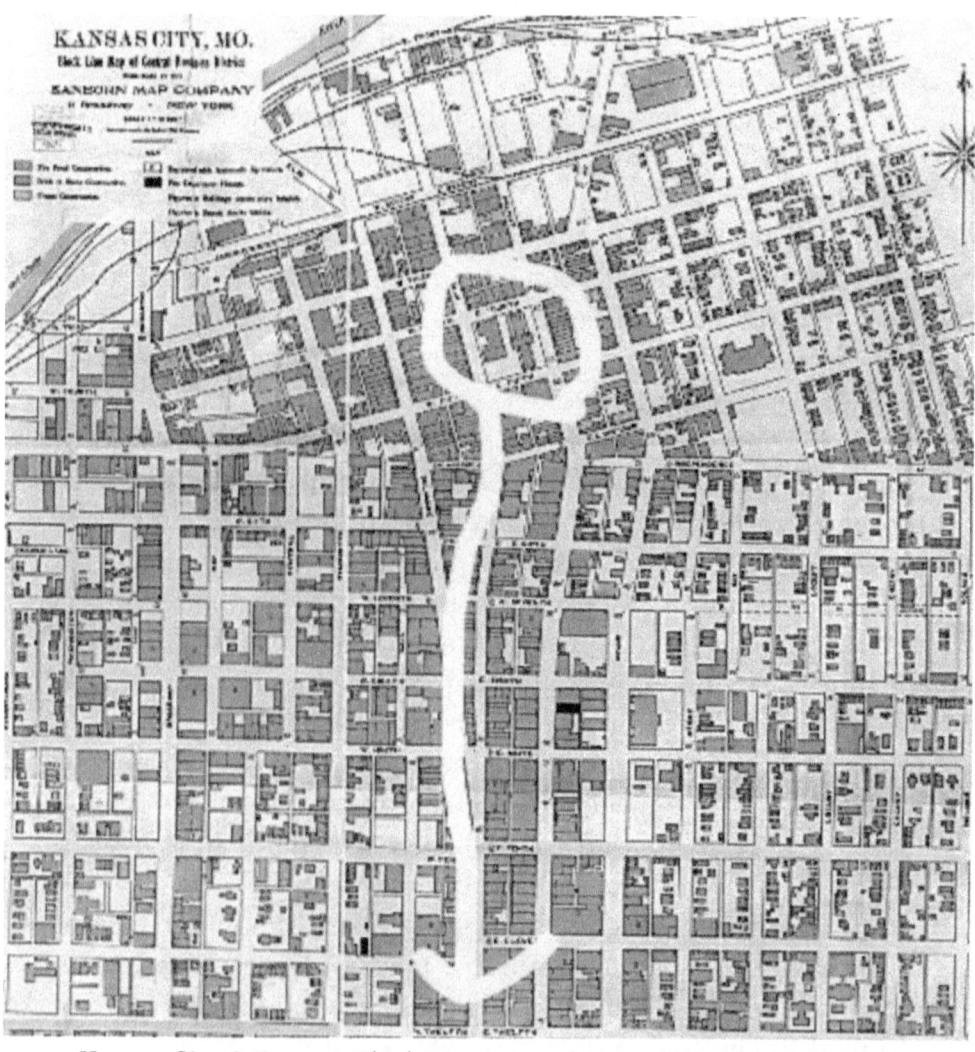

Kansas City, Missouri, Block Line Map of Central Business District," Sanborn Map Company, New York, 1904. Courtesy of the University of Missouri, MU Libraries. The white circle surrounds the City Hall and the arrow points south to the Kansas City General Hospital.

As the interns admitted the three new patients to the meningitis ward of Kansas City General Hospital on Saturday, January 27, 1912, Curtis E. Greenwood, who had been admitted two days previously, died there.[52] The Englishman, Jack Williams, succumbed on Sunday, January 28, 1912.[53] Mr. Greenwood and Mr. Williams were buried at Forest Hill Cemetery[52] and Leeds Cemetery[32] in Kansas City, respectively.

On Tuesday, January 30, 1912, train station personnel called an ambulance to transport a thirty-one-year-old man named William Holt from the Grand Central Train Depot in Kansas City. He had arrived in Kansas City from Texas the day before. Kansas City General Hospital physicians admitted him to the meningitis ward,[54] thereby bringing the number of new cases (from Thursday, January 25, 1912, to Tuesday, January 30, 1912) to six (i.e., Greenwood, Williams, Holt, Carroll, Davis, and Griffin). Dr. Wheeler dispatched sanitary workers to fumigate and disinfect any rooming house that had been the residence of a patient diagnosed with cerebrospinal meningitis. Because of the bitterly cold weather, Dr. Wheeler reopened the rooming houses after fumigation; he did not want the transients to freeze to death outside. He did permanently shutter the Swan House at 528 Main Street in response to a police department request; the Swan House was located across the street from City Hall, which contained the police department.

At least one resident of Kansas City died of cerebrospinal meningitis in another city in January 1912. On Wednesday, January 31, 1912, twenty-seven-year-old Louis Martin Boppert,[55] a railroad auditor with the Missouri Pacific Railway, died of cerebrospinal meningitis during a business trip to Hiawatha, Brown County, Kansas.[56] Six days before his death, he had traveled the ninety miles from Kansas City to Hiawatha to orient a new depot agent. Mr. Boppert had felt ill that same afternoon; checked into the Moreland Hotel in Hiawatha; and called Dr. Willard Wheeler Nye,[57] a longtime Hiawatha physician, for help. Dr. Nye had examined him and pronounced him ill with the grippe. The next morning (Friday, January 26, 1912), Dr. Nye had found Mr. Boppert unconscious in his hotel bed. Dr. Nye had tentatively diagnosed cerebrospinal meningitis and called Dr. Coral Adelbert Lilly[58] of Atchison, Kansas, to consult. Dr. Lilly had arrived forthwith; examined Mr. Boppert; concurred with Dr. Nye's diagnosis of cerebrospinal meningitis; and called Dr. Andrew Lars Skoog,[59] the head of the department of neurology and psychiatry at the University of Kansas School of Medicine, to consult. Dr. Skoog had arrived on Sunday, January 28, 1912; confirmed the diagnosis; administered Flexner antimeningitis serum to the comatose Mr. Boppert; and quarantined him. Dr. Skoog returned the next day and remained with Mr. Boppert until his death on Tuesday, January 30, 1912. A train transported Mr. Boppert's corpse to St. Louis, Missouri, for burial in the family plot.

At the end of January 1912, Dr. Wheeler counted twelve new cases of cerebrospinal meningitis in Kansas City for the month.[60] All twelve had died.[61] Most of the twelve individuals had received their care in the meningitis ward of the Kansas City General Hospital for the following three reasons: the refusal of most private hospitals[62] in Kansas City to accept meningitis cases; the difficulty of treating patients in their homes; and the honed skills of the interns, attending physicians, nurses, and orderlies in caring for patients with the disease. Dr. Luscher wrote, "The burden of the care of a large share of both the rich and the poor have fallen upon us."[63]

CHAPTER 2 NOTES

1. "And Colder Yet Tonight; P. Connor Expects the Mercury to Go to 15 Below; That Will Break All Records for This Time of the Year—Reached 13 Degrees Below at 6:30 O'clock This Morning," *Kansas City Star*, January 6, 1912, 1; "A Record Month in Illness; The Hospital Already Has Had 250 More Cases Than in December [1911]," *Kansas City Star*, January 26, 1912, 3; and "A Winter to Remember," in Craig Ladwig, *The Star: The First 100 Years* (Kansas City, MO: *Kansas City Star*, 1980), 71.

2. W. S. Wheeler, "Tenement and Lodging Houses," Hospital and Health Board, *Fourth Annual Report of the Hospital and Health Board of Kansas City, Missouri, for Fiscal Year April 17, 1911, to April 15, 1912, Inclusive* (Kansas City, MO: Hospital and Health Board, 1912), 61.

3. A description (January 12, 1912) of the rooming houses in Kansas City said, "[Hundreds of men] have been sleeping in offices, hallways, and on chairs and tables in the lodging houses on the North Side. And they are happy to have even such accommodations. The front room of the Swan House (528 Main Street) at night resembles a sheep fold, with the men lying so closely together that not a hand could be passed between. Last night 50 men slept on the floor of the room, which is about 13 feet square. In the center of the room are some small pine tables; men sleep beneath them and two men lie on the table. Propped up in each corner of the room a man is sitting like a guard. To pass from one part of the room to another it is first necessary to ask the men in the way to sit up to give you foot room ... Even though the beds are hard, there is one advantage. Large coal stoves are in the room and these are generally kept nearly at a red heat." "Happy with Floors as Beds: Homeless Men of the North Side Take No Thought of the Morrow," *Kansas City Star*, January 12, 1912, 4.

4. "Cynthia M. Green Dead," *Kansas City Star*, January 7, 1912, 5.

5. "From Meningitis, 55 Die; An Expert Called to Investigate Epidemic at Waco, Tex., All the Fatalities in the Last 25 Days and There Are New 29 Active Cases—Schools and Theater Closed—One Death in Austin," *Kansas City Star*, January 8, 1912, 3.

6. Hospital and Health Board, *Fourth Annual Report of the Hospital and Health Board of Kansas City, Missouri, for Fiscal Year April*

17, 1911, to April 15, 1912, Inclusive (Kansas City, MO: Hospital and Health Board, 1912), 104.

7. "Few Meningitis Cases Here; Only One Instance of the Epidemic Form Reported Since December 1 [1911]," *Kansas City Star*, January 15, 1912, 1.

8. Dr. William Lucien Gist (1881–1956) was born in Leavenworth, Leavenworth County, Kansas, as the second of the five children of Charles Gist (1857–1942), a farmer, and Lucy Frances Snell (1859–1896). His paternal grandfather, John C. Gist, platted the town of Leavenworth, Kansas. Dr. Gist grew up on his parents' farm and attended the Leavenworth public schools before entering the University Medical College of Kansas City in 1906. After graduation, he worked as an emergency surgeon for the Kansas City Hospital and Health Department and as an assistant administrator for the Kansas City Hospital and Health Board during the cerebrospinal meningitis epidemic in 1912. After leaving the municipal health service, he practiced medicine in Kansas City and was on the staff of St. Joseph Hospital for many years. He returned to the municipal health service in 1920 as the superintendent of the Kansas City General Hospital (1920–1924). He served in the military in the Spanish-American War; in the United States Army Medical Corps during World War I and World War II, reaching the rank of major; and in the Missouri Medical Corps as commanding general. He married Gertrude Claire Aaron (1880–1984) in 1907; they had two children. He died in St. Joseph Hospital of pyelonephritis with septicemia and benign hyperplasia of the prostate; he was seventy-five years old. See "William Lucien Gist, MD," in Walter Barlow Stevens, *Centennial History of Missouri (The Center State); One Hundred Years in the Union, 1820–1921* (St. Louis, MO: S. J. Clarke Publishing Company, 1921), 3:811–12. "City Surgeons Selected; The Emergency Force Is Increased from Six to Nine," *Kansas City Times*, May 30, 1911, 8; "Two Diphtheria Cases at General," *Kansas City Times*, February 25, 1921, 6; and "Dr. W. L. Gist Resigns," *Kansas City Star*, June 21, 1924, 1.

9. The Kansas City prevalence measurement of 1.44 afflicted Kansas City residents per 10,000 Kansas City residents for the defined period in 1911 noted in the text comported well with the interepidemic cerebrospinal meningitis prevalences for New York City (Manhattan and the Bronx) for the years from 1894 to 1903 of 1.18, 1.09, 0.93, 1.20, 1.31, 1.42, 0.97, 0.94, 0.87, and 0.86 afflicted

residents per 10,000 New Yorkers (of Manhattan and the Bronx combined), respectively. These low prevalences represent endemic levels of cerebrospinal meningitis (i.e., the constant occurrence of a disease in a population or geographic area). Charles F. Bolduan, "Cerebrospinal Meningitis from the Standpoint of Public Health," *Medical Times* 36, no. 7 (July 1908): 193; and Miquel Porta, *A Dictionary of Epidemiology* (Oxford, England: Oxford University Press, 2014), 92.

10. William Lucien Gist, "Report on Meningitis," Hospital and Health Board, *Fourth Annual Report of the Hospital and Health Board of Kansas City, Missouri, for Fiscal Year April 17, 1911, to April 15, 1912, Inclusive* (Kansas City, MO: Hospital and Health Board, 1912), 103.

11. The evidence that Dr. Hall and Dr. Sophian communicated with one another on Saturday, January 20, 1912, is in a newspaper article in which Dr. Sophian told a Dallas audience that day the following: "I have only today received from Dr. [Frank Johnson] Hall, an eminent authority, commendation of the suggestion for the vaccination, or use of the [Flexner antimeningitis] serum as a preventive." "So-Called Epidemic Practically Over," *Dallas Morning News*, January 21, 1912, 8.

12. Margaret R. O'Leary and Dennis S. O'Leary, *The Texas Meningitis Epidemic, 1911–1913: Origin of the Meningococcal Vaccine* (Bloomington, IN: iUniverse, 2018).

13. Dr. Albert Ware Nash (1883–1934) was born in Garland, Dallas County, Texas, as one of the thirteen children of Mary Frances Hobbs (1858–1918) and Judge Thomas Fletcher Nash (1850–1908). Judge Nash served on the Dallas County-of-Law Court of the Fourteenth District Court of Dallas County and as a member of the Texas State Legislature (1881–1885). Albert Ware Nash moved from Garland to Dallas (about fifteen miles to the southwest) at the age of nine; graduated from Dallas High School in 1902; and earned his medical degree from Vanderbilt University School of Medicine in Nashville, Davidson County, Tennessee, in 1906. He subsequently served as an intern and the hospital steward at the City Hospital in Dallas (1906–1907) and as the assistant health officer in Dallas (1907–1909) before entering private practice. He married Clara Julian (1888–1910) on July 7, 1909; she died on March 5, 1910. On September 1, 1911, he was appointed as the Dallas City health officer. A month later, his diagnosis of the first case of meningitis in Dallas marked the

beginning of the Texas meningitis epidemic (1911–1913). He served as the Dallas City health officer until 1915, when he resumed private medical practice. During World War I, he was a first lieutenant in the United States Army Medical Corps at Base Camp McArthur, Waco. Other positions he held included the presidency of the Dallas County Medical Society (1912–1913); a professorship of therapeutics at the Baylor University College of Medicine (1909–1913); membership in the Dallas City-County Hospital Board (1922–1934); and the presidency of the medical staff of Saint Paul's Sanitarium. In 1913, he married Rose Emma Nielson (1891–1934), the daytime nurse supervisor at the Dallas City Hospital during the height of the cerebrospinal meningitis epidemic (1912) in that city; they had two children. He suffered a heart attack in November 1932. In July 1933, he resumed his duties as medical director of the International Travelers Assurance Association and opened a restricted medical practice in his home. He died of a second heart attack about two hours after his wife died of a severe throat infection. He was fifty years old. See "Dr. Fisher Retires from City's Service; Has Been City Health Officer for Five Years; Will Be Succeeded Today by Dr. A. W. Nash—Submits Some Recommendations," *Dallas Morning News*, September 1, 1911, 4; "Medical News, Texas," *Journal of the American Medical Association* 57, no. 11 (September 9, 1911): 909; "Dr. Albert Ware Nash," in Ellis Arthur Davis and Edwin H. Grobe, *Encyclopedia of Texas* (Dallas, TX: University of North Texas, 1922), 1:237; "Dallas Doctor and Wife Die within Two Hours Each Other," *Corsicana Semi-Weekly Light* (Corsicana, TX), February 13, 1934, 7; "Double Funeral Services Held," *Galveston Daily News* (Galveston, TX), March 15, 1934, 17; "Deaths," *Texas State Journal of Medicine* 30, no. 2 (June 1934): 135; and *Annual Announcement, Baylor University School of Medicine and School of Pharmacy, Dallas, Texas, 1910–1911* (Dallas, TX: Medical Department of Baylor University, 1910), 8.

14. "City Hospital Is Reserved for Cases; Mayor Directs Removal of Other Patients for Handling Meningitis; Gives Free Treatment; City Furnishes Serum, through Health Department, Patients Unable to Pay for It," *Dallas Morning News*, January 7, 1912, 4.

15. United States Bureau of the Census, "Table 14. Population of the 100 Largest Urban Places: 1910," accessed May 22, 2018, https://www.census.gov/population/www/documentation/twps0027/tab14.txt.

16. "Addresses Doctors at Night Meeting; Dr. Sophian Speaks at Session of Dallas County Medical Society; Situation Not Serious; Declares Presence of One Hundred Cases; No Cause for Alarm—Suggests Immunitization [sic]," *Dallas Morning News*, January 7, 1912, 4.

17. Clemens F. von Pirquet and Béla Schick, *Serum Sickness* (Philadelphia, PA: Williams and Wilkins, 1951); "Communication: Serum Sickness," *Texas State Journal of Medicine* 7, no. 12 (April 1912): 335–36; and Abraham Sophian, *Epidemic Cerebrospinal Meningitis* (St. Louis, MO: C. V. Mosby, 1913), 236–38.

18. "Preparing a Banquet for Sophian and Nash; Dallas to Compliment Doctors for Faithful Services; Dr. Sophian Issues Statement Concerning Antiphylactic Effect of Serum; Physicians' Lunch Club Meets," *Dallas Morning News*, January 28, 1912, 6.

19. In 1913, Dr. Sophian wrote, "The utilization of active immunity as a mean of preventing meningitis has not, I believe, been previously advocated." Abraham Sophian, *Epidemic Cerebrospinal Meningitis* (St. Louis, MO: C. V. Mosby, 1913), 190. Of note, the Research Laboratory of the New York City Board of Health produced many bacteriological vaccines but not a meningococcal vaccine. The reasons for this omission are unknown. See William Hallock Park, "The New Activities of the Research Laboratory of the Department of Health," *Monthly Bulletin of the Department of Health* 1–2 (1911–1912): 57–64.

20. At least two previous American investigators had experimented with the inoculation of heat-killed meningococci material. It is unknown whether Dr. Sophian was aware of them. The first person was thirty-one-year-old Dr. David John Davis (1875–1954), who, in Chicago in 1906, purposefully injected himself with a killed (or semi-killed) meningococcal inoculate to study its blood and clinical effects. He documented his subsequent clinical course. He developed a profound toxemia with headache, slight delirium, vomiting, and temperature elevation to 103 degrees Fahrenheit. His white blood cell count soared to 44,050 per cubic milliliter (an eightfold increase from his baseline) on the third day after inoculation, and his opsonic index reached 2.3 (more than doubled) on the second day before returning to normal on day five after the injection. The second person was Boston-based Dr. Timothy Leary (no relation to the authors), the head of the pathology department at Tufts College Medical Department, who manufactured a killed meningococcal vaccine in January 1908. He gave some vials of it to the British governor of Ghana, who had

requested it for use among Ghanaians to try to control the severe cerebrospinal meningitis epidemic underway in that British colony. See David J. Davis, "Studies in Meningococcus Infections," *Journal of Infectious Diseases* 4, no. 4 (November 15, 1907): 558–681; "David J. Davis Papers, 1913–1955," University Library, University of Illinois at Chicago, accessed January 24, 2018, http://findingaids. library.uic.edu/ead/lhsc/016-01-01-20-02b.html; "Tufts Sends Aid to African Coast; Governor of English Colony Takes Back Vaccine for Meningitis; Disease Now Epidemic among the Natives; Local Laboratory Noted for Its Success in Preparation of Remedy," *Boston Herald*, January 10, 1908, 3; and "Cerebrospinal Meningitis," in David Scott, *Epidemic Disease in Ghana, 1901–1960* (London: Oxford University Press, 1965), 85–119.

21. Dr. Sophian explained to newspaper reporters on Sunday, January 7, 1912, "The old menace to armies was typhoid fever. By immunitization [*sic*] this danger has been eliminated. It can be done with meningitis. A relatively small dose, by inoculation, will prevent the development of a large case later. There will be slight temporary discomfort, maybe temporary disability, but the patient or person treated will be made immune … Immunitization [*sic*] may be secured from immediate administering of an inoculating agent." "Addresses Doctors at Night Meeting; Dr. Sophian Speaks at Session of Dallas County Medical Society; Situation Not Serious; Declares Presence of One Hundred Cases; No Cause for Alarm—Suggests Immunitization [*sic*]," *Dallas Morning News*, January 7, 1912, 4. See also "Expert Visits Cases upon Reaching City; Dr. Sophian Has Begun Study of Local Meningitis Situation; Arrived in Dallas Last Night and Confers with Physicians—State Health Officer Here," *Dallas Morning News*, January 6, 1912, 5.

22. The cause of typhoid fever is the *Salmonella enterica typhi* bacterium. Wartime typhoid fever often killed more soldiers than did combat. Dr. Almroth Edward Wright (1861–1947) originated the heat-killed typhoid vaccine at the Royal Army Medical College in England between 1892 and 1902. See Leonard Colebrook, *Almroth Wright: Provocative Doctor and Thinker* (London: Whitefriars Press, 1954); Clara E. Councell, "War and Infectious Disease," *Public Health Reports* 56, no. 12 (March 21, 1941): 547–73; Almroth Edward Wright, *Vaccine Therapy: Its Administration, Value, and Limitations* (London: Longmans, Green, and Company, 1910), 98, 191; and William Cecil Bosanquet and John William Henry Eyre,

Serum, Vaccines, and Toxines [sic] *in Treatment and Diagnosis* (New York: Funk and Wagnalls Company, 1910), 52–54.

23. Of note, Dr. Almroth Edward Wright attributed his idea for the typhoid vaccine to reading about the success of the cholera and bubonic plague vaccines developed by Russian bacteriologist Waldemar Mordecai Haffkine (1860–1930), who had developed cholera and bubonic plague vaccines in the early 1890s for use in British India. See W. Bulloch, "Waldemar Mordecai Wolff Haffkine," *Journal of Pathology and Bacteriology* 34, no. 2 (1931): 125–29; Selman Waksman, *The Brilliant and Tragic Life of W. M. W. Haffkine: Bacteriologist* (New Brunswick, NJ: Rutgers University Press, 1964); and Barbara J. Hawgood, "Waldemar Mordecai Haffkine, CIE (1860–1930): Prophylactic Vaccination against Cholera and Bubonic Plague in British India," *Journal of Medical Biography* 15, no. 1 (2007): 9–19.

24. "Watch Out for Meningitis; Eight Cases Since January 1 at the General Hospital; Above All, Breathe Fresh Air as a Preventive, a Physician Says—Keep the Living Places Sanitary and Don't Neglect Symptoms," *Kansas City Star*, January 24, 1912, 2.

25. "Into the Room of Dread; An Unexpected Visit to the Meningitis Battle Field; Heroines Heavily Veiled in White Seen by a Visitor in the General Hospital—And the Surprise Spelled a Night's Rest," *Kansas City Star*, February 17, 1912, 2.

26. Dr. John Roberts VanAtta (Van Atta) (1884–1966) was born in Cawker City, Mitchell County, Kansas, to John (?) VanAtta and Mary Eleanor VanAtta (1868–1955). John Roberts VanAtta earned his medical degree from the University of Kansas Medical School in 1911 and subsequently became the Kansas City General Hospital's pathologist (1912–1914). He next performed graduate work at the Mayo Clinic in Rochester, Olmsted County, Minnesota, after which he moved to Albuquerque, Bernalillo County, New Mexico. Once in Albuquerque, he organized the clinical pathology and radiology departments at Presbyterian Hospital and founded the VanAtta Laboratory, New Mexico's first pathology and radiology laboratory. He also helped organize the laboratory of the New Mexico State Department. He married Helen Amanda Sisk (1902–1986) in 1902; they had three children. He died after a short illness in Albuquerque at the age of eighty-two years. See "Doctor's 50 Years' Service Recognized," *Albuquerque Journal*, March 4, 1961, 2; "Dr. VanAtta, Medical Pioneer, Dies at Age 82," *Albuquerque Journal*

(Albuquerque, New Mexico), March 31, 1966, 14; and "The People Honor Dr. VanAtta," *Albuquerque Journal*, April 28, 1966, 5.

27. Dr. VanAtta wrote around April 1912, "Stock typhoid and meningococcic vaccines are made in the laboratory and given to those in constant contact with these diseases." Hospital and Health Board, *Fourth Annual Report of the Hospital and Health Board of Kansas City, Missouri, for Fiscal Year April 17, 1911, to April 15, 1912, Inclusive* (Kansas City, MO: Hospital and Health Board, 1912), 28.

28. Perhaps Dr. Luscher was remembering the Kansas City cerebrospinal meningitis epidemic in 1899. See "Many Cases of Meningitis; Kansas City Physicians Say It's Almost an Epidemic; Death Has Come Quickly in a Majority of Cases—Doctors Expect the Coming of Balmy Weather Will Stop Its Spread," *Kansas City Star*, April 10, 1899, 2.

29. Dr. Darwin Delap (1882–1940) was born in Trinidad, Las Animas County, Colorado, as one of the two sons of Dr. Silas Charles Delap (1846–1931) and Marion Kennedy (1846–1894). He earned his bachelor's degree from the University of Wisconsin in 1906 and his medical degree from Rush Medical College in Chicago, Illinois. He moved to Kansas City to work as an ambulance physician and as a surgeon in the Emergency Hospital in the basement of City Hall (1911–1912). He served on the faculty of the University of Kansas School of Medicine beginning in 1915. He married Elizabeth Peirce (Pierce) (1879–1984) in 1911; they had one child. He died of a stroke at the age of fifty-eight years. See *General Catalogue of the Officers and Graduates of the University of Wisconsin, 1849–1907* (Madison, WI: University Press, 1907), 274; "New Appointments," *Graduate Magazine of the University of Kansas* 14, no. 1 (October 1915): 22; and "Dr. Darwin Delap Rites; Services for Physician Will Be Held Tomorrow Morning," *Kansas City Star*, November 11, 1940, 6.

30. "Another Meningitis Case Here; A Railroad Employee Found Ill with the Disease in a Hotel," *Kansas City Star*, January 24, 1912, 2.

31. "C. H. Sharp," Missouri State Board of Health, Bureau of Vital Statistics, Certificate of Death, File No. 1435, Registered No. 322.

32. The Leeds Cemetery opened in May 1911 and closed in 1934 (the total number of graves was 5,082). It is located southwest of the current location (2018) of the Kansas City Sports Complex. Only a few of the early stakes are still visible. No names or marked grave

sites survive. All that remains is rough, hilly land covered by trees and scrub. See "Leeds Cemetery, Kansas City, Jackson County, Missouri," accessed March 26, 2018, https://www.findagrave.com/cemetery/2261469/leeds-cemetery.

33. "Not a Meningitis Epidemic; Physicians Say, However, the Public Must Be on Guard; Two More Victims Taken to the General Hospital This Morning—Persons Convalescing from Other Diseases Especially Susceptible," *Kansas City Star*, January 25, 1912, 6.

34. Curtis E. Greenwood (1885–1912) was born in Missouri as the youngest of the three children of John H. Greenwood (born in 1852) and Susan Greenwood.

35. "Another Meningitis Death," *Kansas City Star*, January 28, 1912, 4.

36. Establishments licensed to sell Flexner antimeningitis serum (antimeningococcic serum) in the United States as of January 12, 1912, were H. K. Mulford Company (Philadelphia, Pennsylvania); Pasteur Institute of Paris (Paris, France); the Health Department of the City of New York; Swiss Serum and Vaccine Institute (Berne, Switzerland); Farbwerke Vormals Meister, Lucius und Bruning (Hoechst-on-Main, Germany); and E. Merck (Darmstadt, Germany). "Establishments Licensed for the Propagation and Sale of Viruses, Serums, Toxins, and Analogous Products," *Public Health Reports* 27, no. 2 (January 12, 1912): 40–41. See also John Parascandola, "The Public Health Service and the Control of Biologics," *Public Health Reports* 110, no. 6 (November–December 1995): 774–75.

37. Dr. Wheeler said in April 1912 that he had obtained the city's antimeningitis serum from Parke-Davis and Company. See Hospital and Health Board, *Fourth Annual Report of the Hospital and Health Board of Kansas City, Missouri, for Fiscal Year April 17, 1911, to April 15, 1912, Inclusive* (Kansas City, MO: Hospital and Health Board, 1912), 107.

38. The Federal Public Health Service was a bureau of the US Treasury Department. The United States surgeon general presided over the Federal Public Health Service bureau in Washington, DC. The bureau, at the time of the publication of the January 1913 backgrounder article noted in the text, consisted of the following seven divisions: personnel and accounts, foreign and insular quarantine and immigration, domestic (interstate) quarantine and sanitation, sanitary reports and statistics, scientific research, marine hospitals and relief, and miscellaneous. An assistant surgeon general oversaw six divisions (excepting miscellaneous). J. W. Kere, "Organization of

the Federal Public Health Service," *Public Health Reports* 28, no. 3 (January 17, 1913): 117–19.

39. Wade Hampton Frost, "Epidemic Cerebrospinal Meningitis: A Review of Its Etiology, Transmission, and Specific Therapy, with Reference to Public Measures for Its Control," *Public Health Reports* 27, no. 4 (January 26, 1912): 97–121.

40. Dr. Wade Hampton Frost (1880–1938) was born in Marshall, Fauquier County, Virginia, as one of the eight children of Dr. Henry Rutledge Frost Jr. (1839–1917) and Sabra Jane Walker (1839–1917). Wade H. Frost earned his bachelor's and medical degrees from the University of Virginia in 1901 and 1903, respectively. While serving in the United States Public Health Service (1905–1929), he studied water pollution, poliomyelitis, yellow fever, influenza, diphtheria, and tuberculosis. In 1931, he resigned from the public health service to serve full-time as a professor of epidemiology and dean of the Johns Hopkins University School of Hygiene and Public Health (1931–1934). He married Susan Noland Haxall (1876–1965) in 1915; they had one child. He died at the age of fifty-eight years at the Johns Hopkins University Hospital. See Thomas M. Daniel, *Wade Hampton Frost, Pioneer Epidemiologist 1880–1938: Up to the Mountain* (Rochester, NY: University of Rochester Press, 2004); and "Dr. W. H. Frost Dies at Johns Hopkins," *Columbia Record* (Columbia, SC), May 2, 1938, 11.

41. Assistant surgeons in the United States Public Health and Marine Hospital in 1911 earned $1,600 per year; passed assistant surgeons earned $2,000 per year; and surgeons earned $2,500 per year. For more information on the qualifications and performance requirements for each grade, see "Bureau of Public Health and Marine Hospital Service," *Texas State Journal of Medicine* 7, no. 1 (May 1911): 31–32.

42. For a history of the United State Public Health Service, see Ralph Chester Williams, *The United States Public Health Service, 1798–1950* (Washington, DC: Officers Association of the United States Public Health Service, 1951).

43. Wade Hampton Frost, "Epidemic Cerebrospinal Meningitis: A Review of Its Etiology, Transmission, and Specific Therapy, with Reference to Public Measures for Its Control," *Public Health Reports* 27, no. 4 (January 26, 1912): 119–20.

44. Ibid., 120–21.

45. An oral dose of urotropin (hexamethylenamine) splits into formaldehyde and ammonia, which leave the body in the urine (for the most part) but also find their way into the cerebrospinal fluid and the nasal mucous membranes. See "Epidemic Meningitis: Editorial," *Medical Herald* 32, no. 2 (February 1913): 75–77; and Phebe L. DuBois, "Differential Diagnosis and Treatment of Epidemic Cerebrospinal Meningitis," *Journal of the American Medical Association* 60, no. 11 (March 15, 1913): 822.

46. "Meningitis Scare Is Over; The Health Board Has Heard of No New Cases in Thirty-Six Hours," *Kansas City Star*, January 27, 1912, 2.

47. "Two New Meningitis Cases in Kansas City," *Topeka Daily Capital* (Topeka, KS), January 29, 1912, 3.

48. "Find a New Meningitis Case; H. A. Davis, a Laborer, the Fourth to Be Stricken at a North Side Hotel," *Kansas City Star*, January 28, 1912, 2.

49. The Emergency Hospital in the basement of City Hall provided immediate care for patients in the busy, high-density north side of Kansas City on the Missouri River. The Emergency Hospital was opened because the Kansas City Municipal Hospital and the Kansas City General Hospital lay twenty blocks south of City Hall. The Emergency Hospital in 1912 consisted of six rooms: a four-cot women's ward, an eight-cot men's ward, a padded detention room, a dispensary, a surgeon's room, and a reception room for patients' friends and relatives. See "Police Headquarters," *Kansas City Star*, December 29, 1906, 4; "An Emergency Hospital, Six Rooms in the City Hall Basement Are to Be Remodeled; Injured Will No Longer Be Carted about the City, but Will Receive Proper Treatment at Once—Four Women Nurses—No Sightseers," *Kansas City Star*, January 10, 1907, 1; "New Emergency Hospital, Improvement Brought about at the City Hall by Dr. Sanders," *Kansas City Star*, April 4, 1907; "A Night with the Police," *Kansas City Star*, April 21, 1907, 14; and "Native Sons and the 'City Fathers' to Discuss Passing of the Old City Hall," *Kansas City Star*, February 28, 1937, 1C, 31.

50. The Kansas City City [*sic*] Hall building in use in 1912 was built in 1892 and was located at the southeast corner of Fourth and Main Street. Police headquarters occupied portions of the first and second floors, the basement, and the subbasement of City Hall until 1907, when Mayor Henry Mahan Beardsley (1858–1938, served as mayor 1906–1907) and Dr. St. Elmo Sanders (1873–1931), the city physician of Kansas City, remodeled the health department rooms in

the south part of City Hall's basement into an Emergency Hospital. See "Police Headquarters," *Kansas City Star*, December 29, 1906, 4; "An Emergency Hospital, Six Rooms in the City Hall Basement Are to Be Remodeled; Injured Will No Longer Be Carted about the City, but Will Receive Proper Treatment at Once—Four Women Nurses—No Sightseers," *Kansas City Star*, January 10, 1907, 1; "New Emergency Hospital, Improvement Brought about at the City Hall by Dr. Sanders," *Kansas City Star*, April 4, 1907; "A Night with the Police," *Kansas City Star*, April 21, 1907, 14; and "Native Sons and the 'City Fathers' to Discuss Passing of the Old City Hall," *Kansas City Star*, February 28, 1937, 1C, 31.

51. Leo Thomas Griffin (1892–1929) was born in Kansas City, Kansas, as a child of Maurice "Morris" Griffin (1862–1908) and Catherine Ann Tooey (1862–1951).

52. "Curtis E. Greenwood," Missouri State Board of Health, Bureau of Vital Statistics, Certificate of Death, File No. 1420, Registered No. 307.

53. "Jack Williams," Missouri State Board of Health, Bureau of Vital Statistics, Certificate of Death, File No. 1439, Registered No. 326.

54. "From Texas with Meningitis; A Man Found at the Grand Central Depot Makes Nine Cases at the Hospital," *Kansas City Star*, January 31, 1912, 10.

55. Louis Martin Boppert (1885–1912) was born in St. Louis, St. Louis County, Missouri, as the younger of the two children of Louis Boppert (1856–1886), a gardener, and Margaret E. Wagner (1861–1951). He worked for the Missouri Pacific Railway for many years.

56. "Kansas City Man Dies of Spinal Meningitis; Was Taken Sick at Hiawatha and Died There Shortly Afterwards," *Kansas City Star*, January 31, 1912, 3; "A Railway Man Dead of Meningitis," *Kansas City Star*, January 31, 1912, 1; "Deaths," *Brown County World* (Hiawatha, KS), February 2, 1912, 2; "Auditor Had Spinal Meningitis," *Kansas Democrat*, February 1, 1912, 1; and "Fatal in Three Days," *Abilene Daily Reflector* (Abilene, KS), January 31, 1912, 1.

57. Dr. Willard Wheeler Nye (1846–1938) was born in Bangor, Penobscot County, Maine, as the eldest of the four children of Elisha Nye (1817–1875), a joiner, and Charlotte Crosby Thomas (1824–1858). At the age of seventeen years, he fought with the Eighth Regiment Kansas Volunteer Infantry for most of the American Civil War. In 1877, he earned his medical degree at Jefferson College in Philadelphia.

In 1879, he moved to Hiawatha, Brown County, Kansas, where he opened a medical a practice and served as the Brown County physician and health officer for decades. He married Margaret Jean McChesney (1851–1949) in 1873; they had three children. He died in Hiawatha at the age of ninety-two years. See "Personal," *Atchison Daily Champion* (Atchison, KS), October 4, 1878, 2; and "Dr. W. W. Nye Named County Physician Again," *Brown County World* (Hiawatha, KS), July 16, 1920, 1.

58. Dr. Coral Adelbert Lilly (1877–1940) was born in Richmond County, Ohio, as a child of Stephen Lilly (born in 1849), a farmer, and Clarissa Baird (born in 1849). He earned his medical degree from Rush Medical College in Chicago, Illinois, in 1901; married Isabel Smith (1875–1925) in 1902; opened a medical practice in Sabetha, Brown County, Kansas; studied medicine in Europe in 1904; and returned to Kansas to open a practice in medicine in Atchison, Atchison County, Kansas. He became a division surgeon for the Missouri Pacific Railway in 1908. In 1927, he attempted suicide by cutting his left palm. He recovered and moved to Michigan, where he taught classes in a Battle Creek hospital and subsequently became a research fellow in the study of rickets and nutrition at the University of Michigan in Ann Arbor, Michigan (1931–1940). He died of a ruptured aorta at the age of sixty-two in Ann Arbor, Washtenaw County, Michigan. See "Social and Personal," *Brown County World*, June 28, 1901, 20; "About Kansas and Kansans," *Independence Daily Reporter* (Independence, KS), August 1, 1904, 1; "Dr. C. A. Lilly, Michigan Dental Researcher, Dies," *Chicago Tribune*, May 5, 1940, 32; "Atchison Doctor Tries to End Own Life in K. C.," *Hutchinson News* (Hutchinson, KS), May 23, 1927, 2.

59. Dr. Andrew Lars Skoog (1877–1960) was born in Carver County, Minnesota, as one of the six children of Johanes (John) Larsson Skoog (1847–1920), a carpenter, and Augusta Charlotte Borg (1855–1949). After earning his medical degree from Northwestern University Medical School in Chicago, Illinois, in 1902, he studied medicine in Europe under Dr. Sigmund Freud (1856–1939) and Dr. Carl Gustav Jung (1875–1961), both of Vienna, and Sir William Gowers (1845–1915) in London. Dr. Skoog was a professor and head of the department of neurology and psychiatry at the University of Kansas from 1908 to 1928. He then left the university to practice medicine in Kansas City until 1955, when he moved to California. He married Anna B. Gordon (1886–1966) in 1910; they had one

child. Dr. Skoog was struck and killed by a car while crossing a street in South Pasadena, Los Angeles County, California, in 1960. He was eighty-three years old. See "Andrew L. Skoog, Psychiatrist Is Fatally Injured in California; California Accident Victim Headed K. U. Department Besides Practicing," *Kansas City Times*, February 6, 1960, 14.

60. Hospital and Health Board, "Contagious Disease Cases Reported for the Year 1911–1912," *Fourth Annual Report of the Hospital and Health Board of Kansas City, Missouri, for Fiscal Year April 17, 1911, to April 15, 1912, Inclusive* (Kansas City, MO: Hospital and Health Board, 1912), 150.

61. Hospital and Health Board, "Contagious and Infectious Diseases Reported; Number and Deaths," *Monthly Report of the Hospital and Health Board, Kansas City, Missouri* 6, no. 1 (January 1912).

62. In 1909, Kansas City had two public hospitals—the Kansas City General Hospital and the Kansas City General Hospital No. 2—and seven private hospitals: the University Hospital (75 beds), owned by the University Medical College of Kansas City at Tenth and Campbell Streets; St. Joseph Hospital (110 beds), founded in 1875 by the Sisters of St. Joseph at Seventh and Pennsylvania Streets; St. Luke's Hospital (25 beds), owned by the Church Charity Association of Kansas City, an organization of the Episcopal Church, and founded in 1882 at 2011 East Eleventh Street; the German Hospital (65 beds), founded by the German Society in 1886 at Twenty-Third and Holmes Streets; South Side Hospital (36 beds) founded by Dr. Laura Payon Hulme (1860–1925) in 1905 at 3007 Main Street; the Red Cross Hospital (20 beds), founded by Dr. Alberta F. Moffet in 1902; and two railroad hospitals, one owned by the Missouri Pacific Railway (30 beds for employees) and the other by the Kansas City Southern Railroad (25 beds for employees). The two railroad hospitals were located at 706 West Tenth Street and 812 Harrison Street, respectively. See John Punton, "Hospitals of Kansas City," in D. M. Bone, *Kansas City Annual, 1907* (Kansas City, MO: Bishop Press, 1906), 61–64.

63. "Report of Superintendent of Hospitals: Cerebrospinal Meningitis," Hospital and Health Board, *Fourth Annual Report of the Hospital and Health Board of Kansas City, Missouri, for Fiscal Year April 17, 1911, to April 15, 1912, Inclusive* (Kansas City, MO: Hospital and Health Board, 1912), 24.

DR. LUSCHER'S "IMAGINITIS," FEBRUARY 1912

On Thursday, February 1, 1912, Dr. Frank Hall of Kansas City joined 250 professional and business notables in the main dining room of the Oriental Hotel in Dallas, Texas, to honor Dr. Abraham Sophian, Dr. Albert Ware Nash, and Dr. Alfred Edward Thayer[1] for their work in combatting the Dallas cerebrospinal meningitis epidemic during January 1912. It is unknown who invited Dr. Hall to this gala. His attendance was not a casual occurrence, as the train trip from Kansas City to Dallas was long—507 miles to the southwest as the crow flies. Someone knew and respected him, as his name headed the alphabetically ordered list of the fifty-five physician banquet attendees.[2]

Dr. Sophian and Dr. Nash have been mentioned earlier in this book (Dr. Sophian, pp. ix, 13, 33n53, 47–49, 57–59; Dr. Nash, pp. 47, 57n13). Dr. Thayer was an academic pathologist on the faculty of the Baylor University College of Medicine, which, at the time, was located in Dallas (1908–1912).[3] When the cerebrospinal meningitis epidemic erupted in Dallas in late December 1911 and early January 1912, Dr. Thayer contacted Dr. Nash to volunteer to examine "the pus or matter taken from the spinal column of patients believed to be suffering from meningitis." Dr. Thayer knew that Dr. Nash advocated the lumbar puncture procedure to obtain cerebrospinal fluid "in every case suspected, so that there may be a proper treatment and not the administration of the serum where it is unnecessary and cannot be beneficial." Dallas taxpayers bore the expense of the microscopic and culture procedures performed by Dr. Thayer and his assistants and medical students.[4]

Dr. Thayer offered his services to Dr. Sophian too after his arrival in Dallas on Friday, January 5, 1912. Dr. Sophian developed a process to identify healthy meningococcal carriers from among Dallas residents exposed to individuals stricken with cerebrospinal meningitis. The process involved the culture of secretions obtained from the nose and throat of healthy contacts. Dr. Thayer sent his medical students, the so-called swabbers, to obtain the samples of nasal and throat secretions from contacts. While Dr. Thayer processed the secretions for the presence of meningococci, workers of the Dallas City Health Department quarantined the swabbed persons and treated them with antiseptic nasal and throat washes. When the results for the presence of meningococci in the secretions were determined to be negative, the Dallas City Health Department lifted the quarantine on the contacts. Dr. Sophian believed this approach was scientific and would check the spread of the disease by healthy carriers.[5-6]

Dr. Thayer worked with Dr. Sophian on a second project. Recall that Dr. Sophian communicated with Dr. Hall on Saturday, January 20, 1912, about manufacturing a heat-killed meningococcal vaccine.[7] Soon after his discussion with Dr. Hall, Dr. Sophian had asked Dr. Thayer to manufacture a meningococcal vaccine.[8] Dr. Thayer had immediately begun to work out the plans for the project.[9] By late January 1912 and early February 1912, Dr. Thayer had manufactured enough heat-killed meningococcal vaccine to vaccinate himself, Dr. Sophian, and other volunteers. All so inoculated denied any harmful or even inconvenient aftereffects.[9] In late January 1912 and early February 1912, Drs. Thayer and Sophian emphatically cautioned publicly that they could not yet accept the vaccine as beyond the experimental stage but expressed optimism that the vaccine would prove itself when there was time to conduct a clinical trial.[8-9]

Dr. Thayer employed three doses of heat-killed meningococci, injected subcutaneously, in his immunization procedure. The first dose contained 500,000,000 (five hundred million) heat-killed meningococci. The second and third doses contained 1,000,000,000 (one thousand million, or one billion) heat-killed meningococci. He administered the second and third doses at intervals of a week to ten days.[9]

It is plausible that Dr. Hall visited Dr. Thayer's laboratory in Dallas to observe his technique of manufacturing a heat-killed meningococcal vaccine.[10] Indeed, the visit to Dr. Thayer's laboratory might have been Dr. Hall's primary reason for traveling to Dallas in the middle of winter during a killer cerebrospinal meningitis epidemic.

Following the Dallas banquet on Thursday, February 1, 1912, Dr. Sophian spent the next week traveling throughout Texas to educate medical audiences on cerebrospinal meningitis. During this tour, he predicted to at least one audience that the cerebrospinal meningitis epidemic in Texas had run its course and would quickly end. He based his prediction on the "history of all meningitis epidemics of this kind, [which] flourish for about three months and then very abruptly disappear."[11] After his lecture tour, Dr. Sophian returned to New York City, believing he had completed his work in Texas.

Dr. Hall returned to Kansas City, where the cerebrospinal meningitis epidemic was accelerating. Dr. Luscher was admitting an average of one person per day to the meningitis ward of the Kansas City General Hospital.[12] For example, on Thursday, February 1, 1912, a Kansas City policeman transported an unconscious male lying on Tenth Street[13] to the Emergency Hospital in the basement of City Hall. Dr. Eugene Adelbert Pond[14] examined him, suspected cerebrospinal meningitis, and sent him to Kansas City General Hospital. On the morning of the unconscious man's admission, Dr. Luscher announced, "I have little hope for the man. He remains unconscious and the disease had made much headway when he came here. It is probable he will die. His is the tenth case now in our isolation ward. Practically all of these have come from cheap hotels and crowded lodging houses. As long as the cases are entirely confined to such places, I see no cause for fear from the disease."[13]

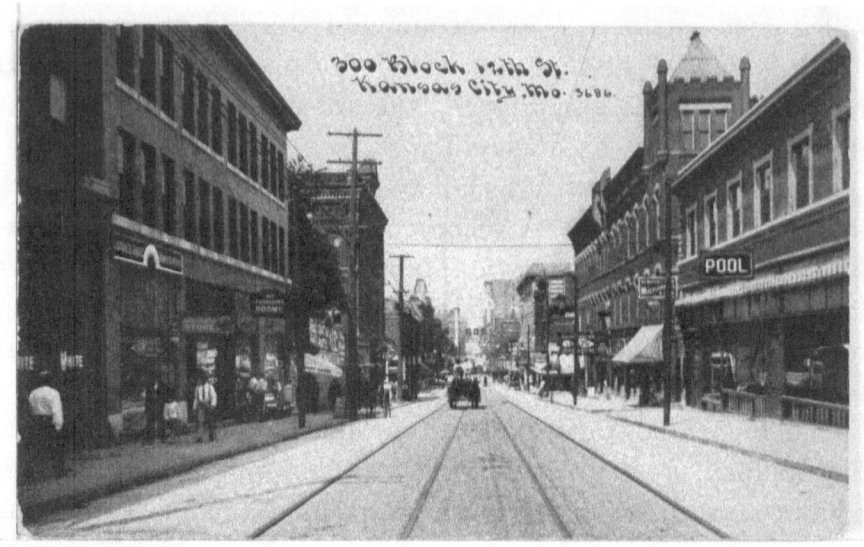

"Postcard of 12th Street at the 300 block and facing east," Kansas City, Missouri, 1909. Vintage postcard is from Mrs. Sam Ray Postcard Collection (SC58), donated to the Missouri Valley Special Collections, Kansas City, Missouri. Courtesy of the Missouri Valley Special Collections, Kansas City, Missouri.

Unfortunately, the disease already had spilled out of the cheap hotels on the north side of Kansas City and into the residential districts of the city. For example, on Friday, February 2, 1912, two sets of brothers simultaneously developed the disease.[12] One set of brothers was eleven-year-old George Frederick Linde Jr.[15] and seven-year-old Canna Simmon Linde.[16] Dr. Wheeler declared on the morning of Friday, February 2, 1912, "These isolated cases in different parts of the city do not indicate a dangerous spread of the disease in any way and should not be taken as indicative of an epidemic. There is no necessity of closing schools where the cases have broken out and there will be no change in daily routine at the schools."[12]

Dr. Wheeler blamed the contraction of the disease by some people on their poor physical condition. People in better health, he said, could encounter "an infected zone" and not contract the disease. He pointed to twenty-seven-year-old Louis Mitchell, a newly admitted patient to the meningitis ward of the Kansas City General Hospital, saying, "The fact that Mitchell lives in a residential district and not in some cheap lodging place in the North Side, as nearly all of our other patients have, is significant. But I hardly believe it indicates any spread of the disease. He may have been in a condition to be infected with the germs."[12]

The next day, Saturday, February 3, 1912, Dr. Frank Chaffee Neff,[17] a Kansas City pediatrician and a member of the attending staff of the Kansas City General Hospital, diagnosed another child with cerebrospinal meningitis. The same day, an unnamed source told a newspaper reporter, "It is the advice of physicians that one should not become frightened or excited about the prevalence of cerebrospinal meningitis as that only has a tendency to prepare one mentally for attracting the disease." The unnamed source averred that no way existed to ward off the disease, that people should go about their duties naturally and quietly, and that if a person believed he or she had become infected, he or she should consult a reputable doctor immediately and submit to a lumbar puncture procedure.

The same unnamed person noted that recovery from cerebrospinal meningitis depended on the length of time between initial infection and treatment with the antiserum. One would know that one had the disease by a sudden rise in temperature to 101 to 105 degrees Fahrenheit, followed by chills, rigidity of the neck muscles, vomiting, extreme headache, possible delirium, and sensitivity to light. The infection started in the nose and throat and ran from a few days to two weeks. Treatment involved isolation and the intraspinal administration of several doses of antimeningitis serum. Little was known about the germs that produced the disease. All of the cases in the city thus far had been among men or boys, but the disease was not peculiar to them. A woman had been one of the earliest cases at the Kansas City General Hospital;

she had died. The Kansas City General Hospital meningitis ward currently contained thirteen patients; nine were getting over the "bad stages" of the disease, and the remaining four had recently been taken into the meningitis ward.[18]

On Sunday, February 4, 1912, the *Kansas City Star* reported thirteen patients with cerebrospinal meningitis in the meningitis ward of the Kansas City General Hospital and five afflicted children receiving treatment in their homes.[19] All were making good progress. There were no new cases that day. The same newspaper article corrected the assertion from the previous day (i.e., that "no way existed to ward off the disease"). Indeed, the article cited Dr. Sophian's recommendation of a nose and throat cleansing with one part of hydrogen peroxide in three parts of water, followed by a spray of menthol gum camphor and liquid alboline (mineral oil). An hour after each meal, Dr. Sophian also advised individuals to swallow a five-grain dose of urotropin dissolved in water.[19]

On Tuesday, February 6, 1912, nineteen-year-old George Beckwith was admitted to the meningitis ward of the Kansas City General Hospital at the same time that twenty-two-year-old George Potter, a married cook, was wheeled out of the ward on his way to the morgue in the hospital basement. Mr. Potter was the eleventh person to die from cerebrospinal meningitis at the Kansas City General Hospital since Monday, January 1, 1912.[20]

On Thursday afternoon, February 8, 1912, Dr. Wheeler received reports of three new cases of cerebrospinal meningitis.[21] The first was an unidentified man found unconscious at around ten o'clock in the morning in a rooming house at 305 1/2 East Twelfth Street. He had entered the rooming house the day before but had not signed the register and had left no means of identification in his room. He died around one o'clock in the afternoon of the same day as his admission to the Kansas City General Hospital.[22]

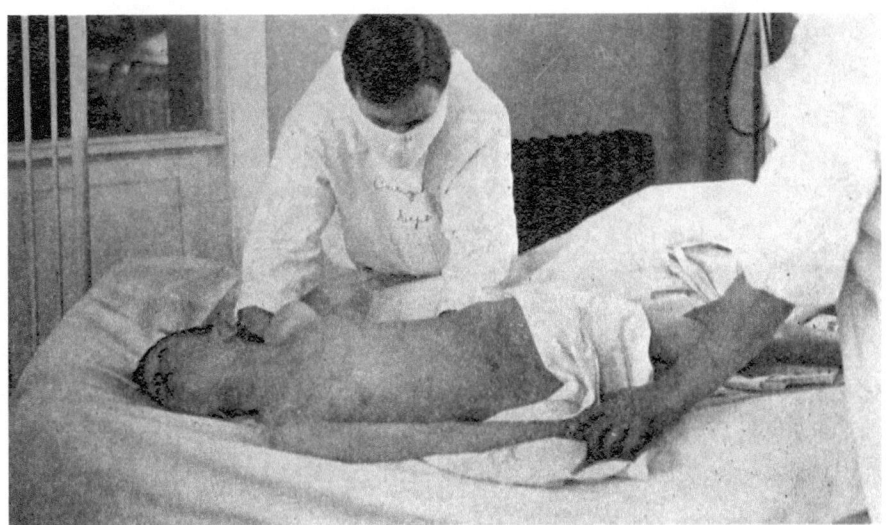

Boy with meningitis, circa 1912–1913. The original caption of this image was: "Boy of eleven, ill forty-eight hours with epidemic meningitis. He was actively delirious so that he had to be held for the photograph. Note the posture. The head markedly retraced, back bowed." The photographer is unknown. Date: circa 1912–1913. The image was scanned from Abraham Sophian, *Epidemic Cerebrospinal Meningitis* (St. Louis, MO: C. V. Mosby, 1913), 73.

The second victim admitted to the meningitis ward of the Kansas City General Hospital on February 8, 1912, was forty-four-year-old Mrs. George Frederick Linde,[23] the mother of George Frederick Linde Jr. and Canna Simmon Linde, the two brothers who had become ill with the disease on Friday, February 2, 1912.[12] Mrs. Linde was dangerously ill at the time of her admission.[21] Her two sons were already receiving their care in the meningitis ward of the Kansas City General Hospital when their mother arrived.

The third victim admitted to the meningitis ward of the Kansas City General Hospital on February 8, 1912, was Thomas Kellogg, a twenty-four-year-old bookkeeper found ill in his bed at the Stag House at about eight thirty the same morning.[12] He had lived in the rooming house for about ten days. His condition was not considered dangerous.[21]

Also, on Thursday, February 8, 1912, five-year-old John Francis Cronin Jr.[24] died of cerebrospinal meningitis in his home in Kansas City at around four o'clock in the morning.[25] Dr. Bertan Wheeler[26] had provided the child's medical care. On Friday, February 9, 1912, thirty-two-year-old Walter Walton, a baggageman who lived at 559 Grand Avenue, Kansas City, was admitted to the Old Hospital for treatment of his cerebrospinal meningitis.[25]

On Saturday, February 10, 1912, an ambulance transported thirty-three-year-old Fred E. Goldsberry, a bookkeeper for the Elite Post Card Company, from 1512 Elmwood Street to the meningitis ward of the Kansas City General Hospital. Hospital physicians diagnosed him with cerebrospinal meningitis and graded his condition as dangerous. Another patient, twenty-year-old Joe Gutirez [sic], a Mexican laborer, also entered the meningitis ward that same day. Physicians graded his condition too as dangerous. The same day, February 10, 1912, thirty-five-year-old John Watson died at the Kansas City General Hospital, where he had struggled with cerebrospinal meningitis since his admission Friday, February 2, 1912. On February 10, 1912, there were fourteen patients with cerebrospinal meningitis under the care of physicians in the meningitis ward of the Kansas City General Hospital.[27]

Sunday, February 11, 1912, passed without a report of a new case of cerebrospinal meningitis in Kansas City. Then, on Monday, February 12, 1912, Dr. Wheeler received reports of four new afflicted individuals:[28] a child of Emmett Martin Ditzler, a roofer;[29] twenty-five-year-old Myron Loewen, a stove manufacturer;[30] twenty-nine-year-old Frank Hunnewell (Hunneywell, Honeywell), an ice wagon driver; and fifty-year-old Mrs. H. Levine. Only Frank Hunnewell received his care at the Kansas City General Hospital. The other three victims were treated in their homes. As of Monday, February 12, 1912, the meningitis ward of the Kansas City General Hospital contained thirteen patients, with several in a dangerous condition.[28]

On Tuesday, February 13, 1912, forty-four-year-old Ira Grant Hedrick,[31] a nationally known civil engineer who resided in Kansas City, developed a severe headache. He called his personal physician, Dr. E. Albert Lieberman,[32] who evaluated him, suspected cerebrospinal meningitis, performed a lumbar puncture procedure, and identified meningococci in Mr. Hedrick's cerebrospinal fluid. Dr. Lieberman administered intraspinal Flexner antimeningitis serum and continued to care for Mr. Hedrick in his home.[33] Mr. Hedrick was certain he had contracted his meningitis in Dallas, Texas, where, two weeks earlier, he had been overseeing construction of the Oak Cliff Viaduct[34] across the Trinity River. When he had returned to Kansas City, he had told Dr. Lieberman, "I am afraid of the disease. I know I am going to become infected." Dr. Lieberman had examined him at that time, pronounced him healthy, and tried to soothe his fears. Mr. Hedrick had visited Dr. Lieberman several more times. When Mr. Hedrick did develop cerebrospinal meningitis two weeks after his return from Dallas, Dr. Lieberman attributed the illness in part to Mr. Hedrick's "highly apprehensive mental condition," noting that "such a mental condition rather attracts the infection and prepares the body for receiving rather than warding off the disease."[33]

Also, on Tuesday, February 13, 1912, a Topeka newspaper reported eight new cases of cerebrospinal meningitis in Kansas City, with five deaths from the disease since Saturday, February 10, 1912. The newspaper also broadcast that one patient was teetering on the edge of death at the Kansas City General Hospital and that two other patients were struggling in critical condition.[35] The Jackson County (Missouri) Medical Society, in the same article, proclaimed that the prevalence of cerebrospinal meningitis in the region was sufficient to call it an epidemic.[35] This newspaper article stoked fear in the Kanas City population.

The next day, Wednesday, February 14, 1912, Dr. Wheeler publicly rebuked the Jackson County Medical Society for indicating that the prevalence of cerebrospinal meningitis was sufficient to call it an epidemic. He declared that there was no epidemic of cerebrospinal meningitis in Kansas City.[36] To prove his point, he compared the number of cerebrospinal meningitis deaths (forty-six) to date (January 1, 1912, to February 14, 1912) in Kansas City to the number of deaths from cerebrospinal meningitis to date in

Dallas (ninety-nine), Fort Worth (fourteen), and Waco (forty-two), noting that the three Texas cities had much smaller populations than Kansas City. Dr. Wheeler said, "[The people of Kansas City] should not be scared."[36]

Also, on Wednesday, February 14, 1912, thirty-nine-year-old Mrs. Effie Sloan Adamson,[37] a professional nurse, was admitted to the meningitis ward of the Kansas City General Hospital. Since Friday, February 1, 1912, she had provided care in the home of eleven-year-old Kurt Ernst Rau and seven-year-old Herbert Rau,[38] two brothers with cerebrospinal meningitis.[39] The presence of a nurse as a patient in the meningitis ward was unnerving to some of the staff members working at the Kansas City General Hospital.

On Thursday, February 15, 1912, the Kansas City Health Department received a report of one new case of cerebrospinal meningitis: six-year-old Joseph Klomp, whose father, Henry Klomp, a laborer in a wholesale house, had called a physician for help when he found his son convulsing at home.[40] The physician sent the dangerously ill child to the Kansas City General Hospital.[41]

On Friday, February 16, 1912, there were no new reports of cerebrospinal meningitis. During the lull, a *Kansas City Star* reporter interviewed Dr. Luscher about the history and treatment of cerebrospinal meningitis. Dr. Luscher provided the following information: The disease dated to 1803 [sic], when Dr. Danielson, "an old practitioner of the War of 1812 days," first recognized and wrote about it. A century earlier, doctors knew scarcely anything about the disease. Now doctors knew that the diplococcus caused cerebrospinal meningitis and that the germ worked its way into the cellular spaces between the meninges, or linings, of the spinal cord and the base of the brain.[42]

Dr. Luscher further explained to the reporter that Dr. Simon Flexner of the Rockefeller Institute in New York City had conducted the first experiments with an antitoxin for the diplococcus, which he had injected into monkeys previously inoculated with the disease. Dr. Luscher said that clinical tests with the antimeningitis serum on patients stricken with cerebrospinal meningitis had begun in 1908 [sic]. Of 712 stricken people treated with the antimeningitis serum, 488 had recovered. Physicians treating an afflicted patient injected about one-half to one ounce of the serum into the base of the spine after first removing some cerebrospinal fluid to avoid the added volume placing "unnatural pressure on the fluid flowing over the brain." Dr. Luscher added that the treatment received by cerebrospinal meningitis patients at the Kansas City General Hospital was an injection of the antimeningitis serum every twenty-four hours for several days.[42]

Dr. Luscher then took the reporter on a tour of the meningitis ward of the Kansas City General Hospital, where the latter observed physicians, nurses, and orderlies wearing ghostly white garments, full head coverings, and rubber gloves.[43-44] Patients occupied thirteen of the ward's twenty beds. Staff had bound the hands and feet of a few patients to prevent them from tossing about and falling out of their beds. Many of the patients were scarcely conscious. Dr. Luscher told the reporter, "[This] big room is the isolation ward for patients infected with cerebrospinal meningitis. Those masks are to prevent possible infection, but the attendants do not know whether or not they are immune from infection with the deadly germs. They work blindly, as all do in caring for meningitis patients. They are heroes and heroines." The reporter, with terror in his eyes, fled the ward, as Dr. Luscher called after him, saying, "There [is] no cause for fear or [I] would not have admitted [you] to the isolation ward."[44] The reporter's article appeared on page two of the *Kansas City Star* the next day, Saturday, February 17, 1912.[44]

Also, on Saturday, February 17, 1912, thirty-nine-year-old Effie Sloan Adamson[45] (the professional nurse earlier noted) and six-year-old Joseph Klomp[46-47] succumbed to cerebrospinal meningitis at the Kansas City General Hospital.[42] As orderlies moved their corpses to the morgue in the basement, other staff members admitted a new patient: twenty-three-year-old George Grimm, a laborer living at 228 West Third Street.[45] Meanwhile, a fourth patient, Lou Mitchell, a laundress who had been in the meningitis ward since February 2, 1912, teetered on the brink of death.[45] Sylvester Hightower, a twenty-two-year-old African American laborer, was admitted to the Old Hospital on Saturday,

February 17, 1912, as only the second African American known to have the disease in Kansas City in 1912. He survived for five days before dying.[47–48]

A spot of bright news occurred on Sunday, February 18, 1912, when fifteen-year-old George Busher, a messenger boy, received his discharge from the meningitis ward of the Kansas City General Hospital. He had been treated for cerebrospinal meningitis since February 2, 1912.[49] He had recovered from his disease.

On Monday, February 19, 1912, two more laborers entered the meningitis ward of the Kansas City General Hospital: forty-year-old James A. Welch, whom police found ill at the Helping Hand Institute at about one o'clock in the morning, and forty-five-year-old Riley Glore, whom police retrieved from Seventh and Mulberry Streets at two o'clock in the morning.[50] The next day, Tuesday, February 20, 1912, four more individuals with cerebrospinal meningitis were admitted to the Kansas City General Hospital meningitis ward. They were Andrew Cribben, a locomotive engineer, who died in the receiving ward of the hospital one minute after arriving; David Davis; twenty-two-year-old Francisco Ferro; and eight-month-old Harold Dall. The number of patients in the meningitis ward was fifteen that day, of whom physicians predicted only twelve had a chance to live. The remaining three moribund patients had entered the ward with far-advanced disease.[50]

Tuesday, February 20, 1912, passed uneventfully. On Wednesday, February 21, 1912, Rachel Beggs was admitted to Kansas City General Hospital with cerebrospinal meningitis, bringing the number of patients in the ward to sixteen. All but two were doing well.[51] On Thursday, February 22, 1912, an ambulance transported William Campbell from his home to the cerebrospinal meningitis ward of the Kansas City General Hospital, bringing the number in the ward to seventeen patients, only three patients shy of capacity for the ward.[52]

On Thursday, February 22, 1912, the newspaper reporter who had toured the meningitis ward with Dr. Luscher on Friday, February 16, developed a headache. He believed he had cerebrospinal meningitis and requested an urgent visit with Dr.

Luscher. After evaluating him, Dr. Luscher diagnosed the reporter with "imaginitis." Dr. Luscher told the reporter, "You would be surprised to know the number of persons who have come to the hospital during this recent meningitis scare to ask for meningitis treatment, fancying, because they had backaches or headaches, that they were infected. It is the same with a long list of infectious diseases." Dr. Luscher added that imaginitis occurred around the world. For example, he told a story about a child in Borneo who had imagined a cobra had bitten it. "The child came as near dying as anyone I ever saw, but I finally saved its life by convincing it that a reptile it had seen was not a cobra." Dr. Luscher believed that fear of a disease caused imaginitis, which, in turn, if strong enough, could attract disease germs into a healthy body. "The combination of imaginitis and disease germs is a difficult one to combat and sometimes results fatally," he said. Dr. Luscher advised the reporter to take good care of himself and busy his mind with wholesome, pleasant thoughts. Then there would be little danger of imaginitis.[53]

On Friday, February 23, 1912, both Riley Glore and James A. Welch died of their cerebrospinal meningitis at the Kansas City General Hospital.[54] Two new patients with cerebrospinal meningitis replaced them: eight-year-old Margaret Strohm and Mrs. Inez Potter.[54]

Three days passed without meningitis news in the Kansas City newspapers. On Tuesday, February 27, 1912, Frank White, a twenty-one-year-old African American porter, died of cerebrospinal meningitis in his home.[55] Another victim, David Davis, who had struggled against his cerebrospinal meningitis since February 20, 1912, as noted above, succumbed to the disease on Wednesday, February 28, 1912. As he was wheeled to the morgue, three new afflicted individuals entered the meningitis ward: Jess Ellis, a thirty-eight-year-old laborer from 1312 Summit Street; thirty-seven-year-old F. W. Gordon, a locomotive engineer discovered ill in a room at the corner of Fifth and Walnut Streets; and W. H. Barton, a fifty-nine-year-old laborer found ill at 4503 Belleview Street.[55]

On Wednesday, February 28, 1912, the *Kansas City Star* reported 109 cases of cerebrospinal meningitis, with forty-nine deaths since January 1, 1912. In addition, on February 28, 1912, the meningitis ward of the Kansas City General Hospital contained twenty-four patients.[55] In February 1912, according to Hospital and Health Board data, cerebrospinal meningitis had become the most common contagious disease in Kansas City.[56]

CHAPTER 3 NOTES

1. Dr. Alfred Edward Thayer (1863–1953) was born in Yonkers, Westchester County, New York, as the youngest of the four children of Stephen Howard Thayer Sr. (1810–1890), a lawyer, and Elizabeth Russell Cox (1829–1901). Dr. Thayer attended Barton Academy in Mobile, Mobile County, Alabama; studied for three years at Williams College (1878–1881) in Williamstown, Berkshire County, Massachusetts; earned his medical degree from the College of Physicians and Surgeons of New York City (1884); served a residency at St. Luke's Hospital for two years (1884–1886); traveled to Europe to study microscopy and pathology under Professors Salomon Stricker (1834–1898) and Alexander Kolisko (1857–1918) in Vienna (1887–1888); served a fellowship in pathology at the Johns Hopkins University School of Medicine (1889–1890); taught anatomy at Yale College (1890–1891); and served as a professor of pathology and bacteriology at West Virginia University (1899–1900) in Morgantown. He next joined the fledgling Cornell University Medical College teaching staff in New York City as an assistant instructor in gross pathology (1900–1903), worked as a vital-statistics statistician for the New York City Board of Health, and won a position as an acting assistant surgeon in the United States Marine Hospital Service. In 1902, while at Cornell University Medical College, he published *Compend of Special Pathology* (Philadelphia, PA: P. Blakiston's Son and Company, 1902). It is likely that Dr. Thayer taught Abraham Sophian during Abraham's first year of medical school at Cornell University Medical College (1902–1903). Dr. Thayer left New York City in 1903 to join the pathology department at the University of Texas Medical Branch at Galveston (1903–1907), where he published *Compend of Pathology: General and Special; A Student's Manual in One Volume* (Philadelphia, PA: P. Blakiston's Son and Company, 1906). He worked diligently to identify the cause of yellow fever, believing that its cause was a bacterium. Scientists subsequently determined that a virus was the cause of yellow fever. Dr. Thayer resigned from the University of Texas Medical Branch in Galveston in 1907 because of his wife's deteriorating health and moved to Florida. He subsequently joined the pathology department of Baylor University College of Medicine, which, from 1908 to 1912, was located in Dallas. On July 1, 1912, he left Dallas for Mobile, Mobile County, Alabama, to chair the pathology department of the

University of Alabama Medical Department. He spent the remainder of his career at the University of Alabama, Mobile. He married May Cahoone Kinney (1869–1909) and Elizabeth Carrie Starr (1893–1977); he had no children. He died at the age of ninety years near Mobile, Alabama. See "The University," *Houston Post*, October 4, 1903, 2; "One of Medical Faculty Quits," *Houston Post*, August 13, 1907, 7; *Cactus, University of Texas Yearbook, 1906* (Austin, TX: Von Boeckmann-Jones Company, 1906), 329; "University Notes," *Wheeling Daily Intelligencer* (Wheeling, WV), November 20, 1899, 4; George J. Rice, G. Weldon Tilley, and Peter A. Dysert, "A History of Pathology and Laboratory Medicine at Baylor University Medical Center," *Proceedings of Baylor University Medical Center* 17, no. 1 (January 2004): 42–55; "Medical News, Alabama," *Journal of the American Medical Association* 68, no. 26 (June 29, 1912): 2037; Marilyn Miller Baker, *The History of Pathology in Texas* (Austin, TX: Texas Society of Pathologists, 1996); and Walter Henrik Moursund, *A History of Baylor University, College of Medicine, 1900–1953* (Houston, TX: Gulf Printing Company, 1956), 50, 205.

2. "Gifts Presented to Foes of Meningitis; At Banquet to Drs. Sophian and Nash Citizens Express Appreciation; Win Battle for Dallas; Fight against Disease Has Reduced Death Rate from 62.5 to Less than 25 Percent," *Dallas Morning News*, February 2, 1912, 2.

3. In 1903, the University of Dallas Medical Department merged with Baylor University in Waco, McLennan County, Texas. The name of the new institution (located in Dallas) was Baylor University College of Medicine. See Walter Henrik Moursund, *A History of Baylor University, College of Medicine, 1900–1953* (Houston, TX: Gulf Printing Company, 1956).

4. "Believe Meningitis Situation Improved; Four Deaths and Five New Cases in Dallas Thursday; City Is Disinfecting Streets and Offers to Make Free Pathological Examination for Patients," *Dallas Morning News*, January 5, 1912, 3.

5. On Saturday, January 13, 1912, a team of fourth-year medical students—the swabbers—began to visit all the residences where meningitis had appeared. Each student carried a satchel containing supplies, including microscope slides, sterile swabs in tubes, a flask of sheep's serum glucose broth, a flask of alcohol, an alcohol lamp, petri dishes with adhesive straps, and a notebook. The purpose of the visits was to obtain nose and throat secretion specimens to conduct tests for the presence of meningococci. The medical students were

trained to swab the noses and throats of the contacts, make smears of the specimen on glass slides, inoculate the culture tubes of sheep's serum glucose broth with the ends of the swabs, and return the culture tubes to Dr. Thayer in the Ramseur Science Hall of Baylor University College of Medicine in Dallas. The exposed persons were quarantined in their residences until the tests on their nasal and throat secretions, performed in Dr. Thayer's laboratory, proved that each exposed person was not a carrier of the meningitis germ, as noted in the text. See "'Can Now Control Situation Easily,'—Dr. A. Sophian; Meningitis Expert Says City Now Prepared to Cope with Disease; Force Well Organized; Effectiveness of Treatment and Cooperation of Physicians Improve Conditions—Record for Day," *Dallas Morning News*, January 13, 1912, 3.

6. Rudolph H. Von Ezdorf, "Cerebrospinal Meningitis in Texas," *Public Health Reports* 27, no. 8 (February 23, 1912): 271–72.

7. "So-Called Epidemic Practically Over," *Dallas Morning News*, January 21, 1912, 8.

8. "Dr. Sophian Gives History of Fight," *Dallas Morning News*, February 3, 1912, 13.

9. "Dr. Thayer Discovers Meningitis Vaccine; Dallas Pathologist Announces Results of Experiments; Believed Preventive Method for Successfully Fighting Disease Has Been Found," *Dallas Morning News*, February 23, 1912, 6; and Alfred Edward Thayer, "The Dallas Epidemic of Meningitis; Preliminary Note on the Laboratory Work," *Texas State Journal of Medicine* 7, no. 11 (March 1912): 305–7.

10. Dr. Thayer manufactured his meningococcal vaccine by culturing the combined cerebrospinal fluids of several afflicted Dallas patients (to produce a polyvalent vaccine) in a test tube partially filled with a jelly made of agar (a kind of seaweed), veal broth, and about one-third-diluted sheep serum. He heated the live culture at a temperature slightly less than that of the human body for forty-eight hours. He then tested the live culture for purity (to assure that only meningococci were present). If contaminants were present, he recultured to eliminate them. From a pure culture, he grew massive cultures over a large surface of the same jelly. Forty-eight hours later, he used sterile salt solution to rinse off the pure culture of live meningococci from the surface of the jelly. He next counted meningococci with the aid of a Zeiss counting chamber, using crystal violet as the diluting fluid. After determining the number

of meningococci in a cubic millimeter, he calculated the number in a cubic centimeter and diluted the cubic centimeter with sterile salt solution (0.75 percent) to reduce the number to five hundred million bacteria per cubic centimeter. Up to this point in the process, the meningococci were alive. He next sterilized them at fifty-five degrees Centigrade (131 degrees Fahrenheit) for two hours, made certain the resulting material held no live meningococci by attempting to culture them, and added one-tenth percent carbolic acid to preserve the vaccine. He placed one cubic centimeter (about fifteen drops) of the vaccine into a small glass container, sealed it in the flame of a Bunsen burner, and stored it for use. Dr. Thayer later reduced the temperature to kill the meningococci from fifty-five degrees Centigrade to forty-five degrees Centigrade (113 degrees Fahrenheit) to boost the vaccine's value for prophylaxis. The entire process of manufacturing a meningococcal vaccine took a week to ten days. See "Dr. Thayer Discovers Meningitis Vaccine; Dallas Pathologist Announces Results of Experiments; Believes Preventive Method for Successfully Fighting Disease Has Been Found," *Dallas Morning News*, February 23, 1912, 6; and Albert Edward Thayer, "The Dallas Epidemic of Meningitis; Preliminary Note on the Laboratory Work," *Texas State Journal of Medicine* 7, no. 11 (March 1912): 305–7.

11. "Meningitis Epidemic to End Abruptly Now, Says Sophian; Dr. Flexner's Assistant Speaks to Tarrant County Medical Society—Two New Cases Here," *Fort Worth Star-Telegram* (Fort Worth, TX), February 4, 1912, 8.

12. "Meningitis in 3 Schools; Still No Fear of an Epidemic, However, Health Officials Say," *Kansas City Star*, February 2, 1912, 2.

13. "Meningitis Case on a Street; The Tenth Victim of the Malady at the General Hospital Will Die," *Kansas City Star*, February 1, 1912, 1.

14. Dr. Eugene Adelbert Pond (1880–1944) was born in Fort Scott, Bourbon County, Kansas, as the youngest of the six children of George F. Pond (1844–1911), an insurance agent, and Ann J. Harrington (1844–1924). He earned his teaching degree from the Kansas Normal College in 1898 and his medical degree from the University Medical College of Kansas City in 1909. He worked for several years in the Emergency Hospital in the basement of Kansas City City Hall [sic] after completing medical school and subsequently served for about thirty years as the physician for the Kansas City Stockyards Company and the Commonwealth Aircraft

Company in Kansas City. He married Beulah Ritter Pond (1890–1974) in 1910; they had one child. See *Scalpel: A Year Book of the University Medical College* (Kansas City, MO: Punton-Clark Publishing Company, 1909), 108; and "Dr. Eugene A. Pond Rites; Services Thursday for Stockyards Physician Who Died Monday," *Kansas City Star*, January 11, 1944, 6.

15. George Frederick Linde (born in 1900) was the eldest of the three sons of George Frederick Linde Sr. (1868–1930), a shoemaker, mechanic, and native of Sweden, and Cynthia Matilda Simmon (1868–1912). It is unknown whether he survived his bout with cerebrospinal meningitis.

16. Canna Simmon Linde (1905–1912) was born as the youngest son of George Frederick Linde (1868–1930), a shoemaker, mechanic, and native of Sweden, and Cynthia Matilda Simmon (1868–1912). He died of cerebrospinal meningitis in the Kansas City General Hospital on Sunday, March 3, 1912, after struggling with the disease since Friday, February 2, 1912; he was seven years old.

17. Dr. Frank Chaffee Neff (1872–1947) was born in Winchester, Randolph County, Indiana, as one of the seven children of Ann Hassleton Chaffee (1833–1906) and Andrew Jackson Neff (1825–1904), a boot and shoe merchant and a brevet brigadier general in the American Civil War. Frank Neff attended the University of Iowa before earning his medical degree from the University Medical College of Kansas City in 1897. He worked for one year at the New York Infant Asylum in Manhattan and for two years at the Kings County Hospital in Brooklyn. After eight years of general practice in Kansas City, he studied medicine in Germany. He returned to Kansas City to practice pediatrics for the remainder of his career. He married Helen Josephine Cole (1875–1948); they had three children. See "Frank C. Neff, MD 1872–1947," *American Journal of Diseases of Children* 75, no. 4 (1948), 608–9.

18. "A Child of 3 Has Meningitis, Don't Worry about Getting the Disease, Physicians Advise," *Kansas City Star*, February 3, 1912, 2.

19. "No New Meningitis Cases; The Eighteen Persons Affected Are Reported to Be Making Progress," *Kansas City Star*, February 4, 1912, 9.

20. "One New Meningitis Case; A Boy of 19 Afflicted—The Eleventh Death This Morning," *Kansas City Star*, February 6, 1912, 1. See also "Meningitis Is Spreading, Thirteenth Death from Malady at Durant, Okla; One Patient Dies at Kansas City Last Night and

Another Is Not Expected to Recover," *Ottawa Daily Republic* (Ottawa, KS), February 6, 1912, 1.

21. "Meningitis Fatal to Another; One of Three New Cases Caused [*sic*] Death This Afternoon—A Woman Hit," *Kansas City Star*, February 8, 1912, 2.

22. "A Meningitis Victim Unknown," *Kansas City Star*, February 10, 1912, 2.

23. Mrs. George F. Linde, née Cynthia Matilda Simmon (1868–1912), was born in Rock Island, Rock Island County, Illinois. She married George F. Linde in 1899; bore three children (George F. Jr., Julius, and Canna); and succumbed to cerebrospinal meningitis on Friday, February 23, 1912, after struggling with the disease since Thursday, February 8, 1912. She was forty-four years old when she died. She was buried in her native Rock Island, Illinois.

24. John Francis Cronin Jr. (1906–1912) was one of the eight children of John Francis Cronin Sr. (1873–1929), a salesman for Cudahy Packing Company, one of the Big Four meat packinghouses in Kansas City (Cudahy, Armour, Swift, and Wilson), and Sarah Katherine Carr (1881–1965). His parents gave a son born in 1912 his name, so there were two John Francis Cronin Jrs.: one born in 1906 and one born in 1912.

25. "Meningitis Kills a Boy of 6; A Son of J. F. Cronin Died 20 Hours after an Attack—New North Side Case," *Kansas City Star*, February 9, 1912, 1; and "John Francis Cronin (Jr.)," Missouri State Board of Health Bureau of Vital Statistics Certificate of Death, Registration District 399, File No. 5230, Primary Registration District No. 1002, and Registered No. 445.

26. Dr. Bertan Henry Wheeler (1872–1916) was born in Osborn, DeKalb County, Missouri, as the only child of Henry T. Wheeler (1847–1926) and Marie E. Langren (1852–1927). He earned his medical degree from the Kansas City Medical College in 1894. Dr. Wheeler married Emma G. Gordon (1874–1955); they had three children.

27. "Meningitis Fatal to Another and a New Case Was Reported to the Health Authorities This Morning," *Kansas City Star*, February 10, 1912, 1.

28. "Meningitis Attacks 4 More; One Woman Dead and Several Persons Reported in Danger; There Are Now Thirteen Afflicted with the Cerebrospinal Disease under Treatment in the Isolation Ward at the General Hospital," *Kansas City Star*, February 12, 1912, 4.

29. Emmett Ditzler (1888–1951), a roofer, and his wife, Carrie (1887–1961), had two young sons: Emmett J. Ditzler (1910–1977) and Buford G. Ditzler (1911–1978). It is unknown which of the two sons had cerebrospinal meningitis in 1912; however, he apparently survived.

30. Myron Aaron Loewen (1886–1970) was born in Columbus, Cherokee County, Kansas, as one of the three children of Louis Loewen (1855–1943), a stove manufacturer, and Julia Wisburn (1859–1902). Myron Loewen married Florence Disman (1887–1947), who managed the Vogue Shop. They had no children.

31. Ira Grant Hedrick (1868–1937) was born in West Salem, Edwards County, Illinois, as one of the eight children of Henderson Hedrick (1837–1922), a farmer, and Mary Ann Bryan (1848–1942). He earned a bachelor's degree in engineering from the University of Arkansas at Fayetteville, Washington County, Arkansas, in 1892. He also earned a bachelor of science degree, a master of science degree, and a doctor of science degree from McGill University in Montreal, Canada, in 1898, 1899, and 1900, respectively. After completing his degree at the University of Arkansas, he moved to Kansas City to work as a civil engineer. Between 1907 and 1909, he built the Inter-City Viaduct, which connected Kansas City, Kansas, with Kansas City, Missouri. He also served as the president of the Kansas City Viaduct and Terminal Railway Company. By 1912, he was designing some of the most important engineering works in the United States, including the Red River Bridge in Garland, Miller County, Arkansas, and the Oak Cliff Viaduct in Dallas, Texas. He later designed the Clarendon Bridge spanning the White River at Clarendon, Monroe County, Arkansas, and the Burnside Lift Span in Portland, Multnomah County, Oregon. He married Nancy Louise Luther (1872–1908) in 1889. After her death, he married Malinda Adeline "Addie" Luther (1877–1917) in 1909. After her death, he married Mary Elma Bryan (1881–1974) in 1926. He had three children by his first wife and one child by his second wife. He died in Garland, Arkansas, at the age of sixty-nine years. See "Ira Grant Hedrick," in *Men of Affairs in Greater Kansas City: A Newspaper Reference Work* (Kansas City, MO: Kansas City Press Club, 1912), 106; and "Ira Hedrick, Noted Bridge Builder, Dies," *Arkansas Gazette* (Little Rock, AR), December 29, 1937, 7.

32. Dr. B. Albert Lieberman (1874–1951) was born in Louisville, Jefferson County, Kentucky, as the eldest of the three children of Louis S. (Sam)

Lieberman (1849–1940) and Bertha Mannheimer (1853–1929). He moved to Kansas City as a young boy; graduated from the Central High School in Kansas City (1893); earned a medical degree from the University Medical College of Kansas City; and earned a second medical degree from Bellevue Hospital Medical College in New York City (1896). He returned to Kansas City and opened a general medical practice. He married Beatrice Reefer (1877–1960) in 1904; they had two children. Dr. Lieberman died at the age of seventy-seven years. See W. J. Maxwell, *General Alumni Catalogue of New York University, 1833–1907: Medical Alumni* (New York: General Alumni Society, 1908), 512.

33. "Fear of Meningitis Won; Ira G. Hedrick Stricken after a Visit to Dallas, Tex.; Ever Since His Return He Had Been Apprehensive—Mental Condition Had Much to Do with the Case, Physician Says," *Kansas City Star*, February 13, 1912, 2.

34. The Oak Cliff Viaduct was constructed between 1910 and 1912. At the time of its construction, it was the longest reinforced concrete highway viaduct in the world at 5,106 feet and the first high-level, all-weather crossing of the Trinity River at Dallas. Many previous bridges across the Trinity River had succumbed to flooding. See "Dallas-Oak Cliff Viaduct," *Structurae*, accessed March 22, 2018, https://structurae.net/structures/dallas-oak-cliff-viaduct.

35. "Tell of Epidemic: Meningitis in Kansas City Has Become Serious, Doctors Say," *Topeka State Journal* (Topeka, KS), February 13, 1912, 1.

36. "Meningitis Closes a Kansas School; Action Follow Deaths of Two Children Near Abilene Today; Is Milder at Kansas City; Health Commission Says Disease Is Not Epidemic Although Many Are Yet Stricken with the Malady—Two Deaths Near Salina and the Schools May Close There," *Ottawa Daily Republic*, February 14, 1912, 1.

37. Effie Lucinda Sloan Adamson (1872–1912) was born in Venango, Butler County, Pennsylvania, as one of the sixteen children of George Henry Sloan (1837–1907), a farmer and merchant, and Margaret Adleman (Addleman) (1840–1909). Effie began working as a nurse in Kansas City in 1894. See "A Nurse Takes Meningitis; Mrs. Lou Adamson Was Caring for Two Afflicted Children; Ira G. Hedrick Who Had a Premonition He Would Be Attacked by the Disease, Is Improving—One Other New Case Today," *Kansas City Star*, February 14, 1912, 4; and "Nurse Dies of Meningitis," *Kansas City Star*, February 17, 1912, 1.

38. Kurt Ernst Rau (1900–1972) was born in Solingen, North Rhine-Westphalia, Germany, as the eldest of the three sons of Gus Rau (1872–1931), a contractor, and Anna Rau (born in 1870). He immigrated with his parents to the United States in 1902. His younger brother, Herbert Julius Rau (1904–1978), was born in Cincinnati, Hamilton County, Ohio. Both boys survived their bouts with cerebrospinal meningitis.

39. "A Nurse Takes Meningitis; Mrs. Lou Adamson Was Caring for Two Afflicted Children; Ira G. Hedrick Who Had a Premonition He Would Be Attacked by the Disease, Is Improving—One Other New Case Today," *Kansas City Star*, February 14, 1912, 4.

40. Dr. George A. Graham (1861–1933) was born in Canada. The place of his medical training is unknown. He developed diabetes mellitus and required amputation of both of his legs in 1924. He continued to work, using artificial legs to drive himself in an automobile to his office. He married Ida E. Dailey (1867–1936) in 1887; they had no children. He died of his diabetes at the age of seventy-two years. "Courage Is Infectious," *Kansas City Star*, July 27, 1924, 60.

41. "Meningitis Kills Two More; At the Hospital Sixteen Persons Have Succumbed to the Disease," *Kansas City Star*, February 15, 1912, 1.

42. "Nerve Centers Its Prey; The Meningitis Germ Is an Enemy Science Dreads; Doctors Have Been Unable to Do Much More Than Identify the Diplococcus—The Serum Treatment, but It's Risky," *Kansas City Star*, February 16, 1912, 1.

43. The Kansas City General Hospital staff relied on personal protective equipment—gowns, gloves, head coverings, and masks—to prevent contracting cerebrospinal meningitis from their patients. Jane D. Siegel, Emily Rhinehart, Marguerite Jackson, et al., *Guideline for Isolation Precautions: Preventing Transmission of Infectious Agents in Healthcare Settings (2007)* (Atlanta, GA: Centers for Disease Control and Prevention, 2007): 49–54.

44. "Into the Room of Dread; An Unexpected Visit to the Meningitis Battle Field; Heroines Heavily Veiled in White Seen by a Visitor in the General Hospital—And the Surprise Spelled a Night's Rest," *Kansas City Star*, February 17, 1912, 2.

45. "Nurse Dies of Meningitis," *Kansas City Star*, February 17, 1912, 1.

46. "Joseph Klomp," Missouri State Board of Health Bureau of Vital Statistics Certificate of Death, Registration District 899, File No. 5339, Primary Registration District No. 1002, and Registered No. 554.

47. "Meningitis Fatal to 3 More; Two Children and a Man Die in the Two Kansas Citys—Two New Cases," *Kansas City Star*, February 18, 1912, 2.

48. "Sylvester Hightower," Missouri State Board of Health Bureau of Vital Statistics Certificate of Death, Registration District 399, File No. 5395, Primary Registration District No. 1002, and Registered No. 610.

49. "Two New Meningitis Cases; There Are Still Thirteen Cases in the Isolation Ward at the Hospital," *Kansas City Star*, February 19, 1912, 2.

50. "Four New Meningitis Cases; One Patient Died in a Minute after Reaching the Hospital," *Kansas City Star*, February 20, 1912, 12.

51. "One New Meningitis Case," *Kansas City Star*, February 21, 1912, 12.

52. "Meningitis Attacks One More: William Campbell's Case Makes the Sixteenth Now at the Hospital," *Kansas City Star*, February 22, 1912, 10.

53. "Fear of Illness a Disease; Doctor Luscher Described the Ailment of Imaginitis; It's the Same the World Over, the Hospital Superintendent Tells a Man Who Fancied He Had Meningitis—Keep Your Thoughts Wholesome," *Kansas City Star*, February 22, 1912, 5.

54. "Two Deaths from Meningitis; Health Board Also Hears of Two New Cases Today," *Kansas City Star*, February 23, 1912, 1.

55. "Three New Meningitis Cases; Two More Deaths from the Disease Today, Making Total of Forty-Nine," *Kansas City Star*, February 28, 1912, 2.

56. Hospital and Health Board, "Contagious Disease Cases Reported for the Year 1911–12," *Fourth Annual Report of the Hospital and Health Board of Kansas City, Missouri, for Fiscal Year April 17, 1911, to April 15, 1912, Inclusive* (Kansas City, MO: Hospital and Health Board, 1912), 150.

CHAPTER 4

A DIRE SERUM SHORTAGE, MARCH 1912

On Friday, March 1, 1912, Dr. Wheeler and Dr. Luscher began to grasp the enormity of the worsening cerebrospinal meningitis epidemic. Dr. Wheeler charged Dr. Gist with visiting every rooming house, hotel, and other residences of people stricken with cerebrospinal meningitis for the purpose of causing an immediate cleanup of the premises and a complete disinfection of the room in which each stricken patient had resided.[1]

In addition, between Friday, March 1, 1912, and Monday, March 4, 1912, Dr. Wheeler widely distributed a health department circular to call the public's attention to sanitary measures and the prophylaxis necessary to prevent people from contracting cerebrospinal meningitis. He sent forty thousand of these circulars to the largest employers of labor in the city, whose staff placed them in each employee's weekly pay envelope. From there, the circulars made their way into the homes of the city's population. This was the first time in recent memory, said Dr. Wheeler, that a health emergency had demanded a public circular.[1] The frank advice given by Dr. Wheeler in his circular follows:

> The prevalence of cerebrospinal meningitis in the city and the continued reporting of new cases to the department of health leads the hospital and health

board to believe that it is wise and advisable at this time to issue instructions to the general public concerning the prevention and transmission of this trouble. It is a known fact that fresh air and sunlight prohibit the growth of the germ. Especially do we caution about the ventilation in the home. Do not be afraid to have too much air or light in the room. Do not be afraid to open the windows. Fresh air never killed anybody, but many have died from the want of it. Throw up the blinds and let the sunlight pour into your rooms. Never mind fading carpets and draperies—better they should fade than your cheeks. You cannot get too much fresh air and sunshine, but you can get too little. Throw the doors open at least twice a day and flush the foul air out of the house. You cannot get ventilation through three or four one-inch holes in the storm sash. If you feel cold in the house, do not shut the windows, but put on more clothes and fire. Better to be a little cool and healthy than to breathe dry overheated and foul air, and so lower your vitality and increase your susceptibility to disease.

One of the first steps in the prevention and transmission of this disease is to impress upon the minds of the people that the sanitary laws of the city must be obeyed to the letter; that all deficient plumbing and insufficient toilet equipment should be corrected at once; the back yards [sic] and alleys and outhouses should be placed in a complete sanitary condition, and all garbage and refuse should be removed as promptly as possible.

As the disease is probably transmitted directly from person to person, it is best that no one except nurse or attending physician come in contact with the infected person, and that all excreta be disinfected at once, and everything in the sick room be kept in a cleanly manner. It is deemed advisable, whenever possible, that every case of meningitis be removed to the hospital, where it can be isolated and cared for intelligently, and after the removal of the patient, the house be thoroughly fumigated and disinfected.

As the germ of cerebrospinal meningitis gains its entrance through the nasal and throat passages, it is very essential that these organs be kept in a cleanly condition. This can be accomplished by gargling and rinsing the mouth and cleaning the nose night and morning with some antiseptic solution. In addition to the above treatment, use a stiff tooth brush with a mild antiseptic or dentifrice after each meal. Keep the body and system in as healthy condition as possible; avoid all excesses and BANISH FROM THE MIND ALL FEAR OF THE CONTRACTION OF THIS DISEASE [caps in original].

The health commissioner believes that this brief statement to the public at this time, when so many people are unnecessarily alarmed, will tend to control the fears and assist them in avoiding the contraction of that dreadful disease.

W. S. Wheeler, MD
Health Commissioner[2]

While Dr. Wheeler was composing the above circular, on Friday, March 1, 1912, Mr. Hedrick, the Kansas City civil engineer who had developed cerebrospinal meningitis on February 13, 1912, announced that he was receiving visitors for the first time despite still having a swollen left wrist. His physician said that a swollen, painful joint was a symptom that often followed the disease and that Mr. Hedrick would soon recover from it. The same day, seventeen-year-old Albert Fisher, an employee of the Shukert Fur Company, was admitted to the meningitis ward of the Kansas City General Hospital for treatment of his cerebrospinal meningitis.[3]

Also, on March 1, 1912, three new attending physicians—Dr. Murphy, Dr. Hamilton, and Dr. Child—started their six-month rotation (March 1, 1912, to September 1, 1912) on the wards of the Kansas City General Hospital. They relieved Dr. Robinson, Dr. Lowe, and Dr. Conover, who had served their rotation from September 1, 1911, to March 1, 1912, as noted above.

On Saturday, March 2, 1912, fifty-eight-year-old W. H. Burton died in the Kansas City General Hospital meningitis ward. He had struggled with cerebrospinal meningitis since the previous Monday, February 26, 1912, and left behind a wife and three daughters. He was the ward's fifty-fourth death since Monday, January 1, 1912.[4] On the same day as his death, four new patients were admitted to the meningitis ward: ten-year-old Marie Ennis;[5] a delirious unidentified man about forty-five years old; six-year-old Helen Cain; and forty-four-year-old John Colley, a laborer for the Burlington Railroad, who had been living at the Helping Hand Institute. The number of patients in the isolation ward at midnight on Saturday, March 2, 1912, was twenty-eight.[4]

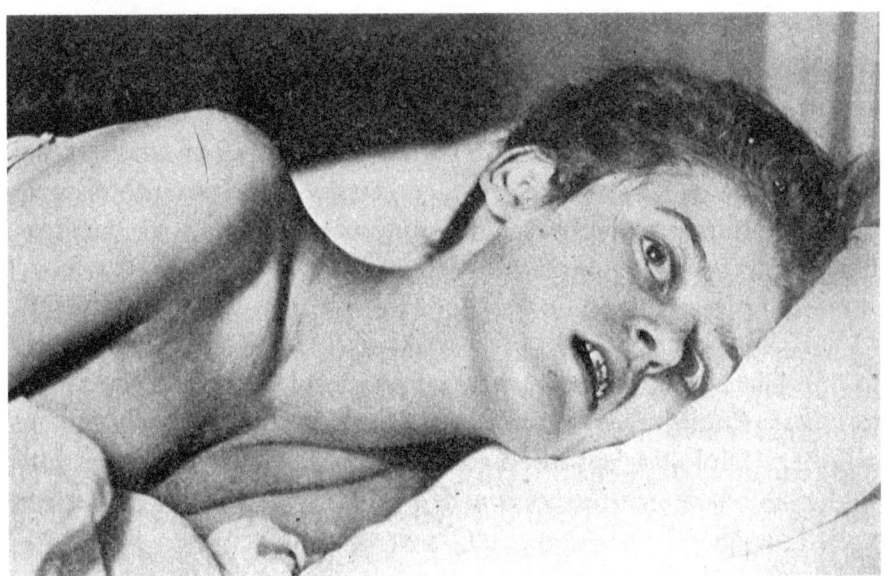

A young girl stricken with cerebrospinal meningitis, 1912. The original caption accompanying this image is: "Patient actively ill six days with epidemic meningitis. She was apathetic but otherwise clear and responded to questions. Note the anxious expression; the retraction of the head; the dilated pupils; the right facial paralysis; right external strabismus, and the sordes on the teeth." The photographer is unknown. The image was scanned from Abraham Sophian, *Epidemic Cerebrospinal Meningitis* (St. Louis, MO: C. V. Mosby, 1913), 72.

On Monday, March 4, 1912, fifty-year-old John B. Watson, a traveler staying at the Lafayette Hotel, was admitted to the Kansas City General Hospital meningitis ward for treatment of his cerebrospinal meningitis. In addition, three African Americans stricken with the disease were admitted to the Old Hospital for treatment. They were seventeen-year-old Eddie Farrell, twelve-year-old Fred Robinson, and twenty-four-year-old General Fayles. Physicians at the Old Hospital were now treating five patients with cerebrospinal meningitis.[6]

On Tuesday, March 5, 1912, ten-year-old Marie Ennis died at the Kansas City General Hospital after her three-day fight against cerebrospinal meningitis.[7-8] The next day, three new patients rolled into the meningitis ward[8]: Mrs. Mary Broom, a patient of Dr. John

Wesley Nixon;[9] forty-two-year-old Mrs. Josephine Fuller; and fifteen-year-old Guy Norton. The latter two individuals, who had far-advanced symptoms of the disease, were not expected to live.[8]

On Thursday, March 7, 1912, Albert Fisher, the Shukert Fur Company employee noted above, and thirty-three-year-old George Grimm, a laborer, died in the meningitis ward of the Kansas City General Hospital.[10] In addition, forty-eight-year-old Reverend Alexander Lewis,[11] the well-known pastor of the Kansas City First Congregational Church, died of cerebrospinal meningitis in his home. On the previous Sunday, March 3, 1912, Reverend Lewis had preached with his usual vigor; on Monday, March 4, 1912, he had read a paper, "The Socialism of Jesus," before the Ministerial Alliance of Kansas City; and, on Tuesday, March 5, 1912, he had performed his usual duties before retiring that evening with a slight headache and a sore throat. He had arisen from his bed about four o'clock on the morning of Wednesday, March 6, 1912, and fallen unconscious to the floor.[12] Dr. William Clay Morris[13] and Dr. Robert Tarleton Sloan[14] had administered Flexner antimeningitis serum by noon on Wednesday, March 6, 1912, but Reverend Lewis died eighteen hours later, never having regained consciousness.[12] Newspapers around the United States reported his death.[15]

Also, on Thursday, March 7, 1912, two new patients were admitted to the meningitis ward of the Kansas City General Hospital: Lenora Dunham, a seven-year-old foundling with advanced disease, and seven-year-old John Wehmeyer. Two other new patients were admitted to the Old Hospital for the treatment of their cerebrospinal meningitis: six-year-old James Hewter and W. H Dawley. Dr. Wheeler responded as follows to the burgeoning number of cerebrospinal meningitis cases in the city: "While we are doing everything possible to combat the disease, I believe that [the] most effective influence against it would be a week of warm, sunshiny weather. With the aid of that we could stamp it out entirely."[17]

As the number of new patients with cerebrospinal meningitis increased between February 22, 1912, and March 7, 1912, the demand for antimeningitis serum increased proportionately.

Kansas City suppliers of the antimeningitis serum could not keep up with the demand for it, which resulted in a shortage. Kansas City physicians and health department officials had been obtaining the antimeningitis serum from two companies—the H. K. Mulford Company and Parke-Davis and Company—since January 1, 1912. On March 7, 1912, H. K. Mulford Company office staff in Kansas City wired their headquarters in Philadelphia to send more serum and promised Kansas City physicians that a new shipment would arrive within a week.[18]

Beginning Friday, March 8, 1912, the *Kansas City Star*, for unknown reasons, sharply curtailed the publication of news about the ongoing cerebrospinal meningitis epidemic. The *Kansas City Star* published one article on Monday, March, 11, 1912, which featured Dr. Luscher encouraging people to go outdoors for fresh air even though the weather was still poor.[19] The next article appeared eleven days later, on Friday, March 22, 1912, when the *Kansas City Star* reported two deaths from meningitis: Mrs. La Rue Duncan, the wife of LaVelle I. Duncan, the sergeant at arms in the lower house of the city council,[20] and Niles Lagerberg.[21] The next newspaper article on meningitis appeared on Saturday, March 23, 1912, announcing the death of fifty-two-year-old Mrs. Mary C. Stafford in the meningitis ward of the Kansas City General Hospital. She had been recovering nicely but died while strolling around the meningitis ward. Her physicians believed she had died of a heart attack.[22] The next day, Sunday, March 24, 1912, forty-two-year-old Mrs. Emma Sisson died in the meningitis ward of the Kansas City General Hospital after a several-day illness.[23] The final *Kansas City Star* meningitis article for the month of March appeared on Sunday, March 31, 1912, notifying readers that sixteen-year-old Katherine Wolfe had died in her home of cerebrospinal meningitis. She had been ill only several hours.[24]

Meanwhile, during the month of March 1912, the Hospital and Health Board reported 113 cases of cerebrospinal meningitis and forty-nine deaths[25] from the disease. The board had received reports of seventy-three cases of cerebrospinal meningitis in February 1912 and twelve cases in January 1912.[26-27] Thus, the total case count of the disease between January 1, 1912, and March 31, 1912, was 198. The prevalence during this same period calculated to *7.92 cerebrospinal meningitis cases per 10,000 Kansas City residents.*

As the Hospital and Health Board digested this grim data, the supply of antimeningitis serum completely ran out in Kansas City on Wednesday, March 27, 1912. For at least four days (until March 31, 1912, and probably longer), not a single dose of antimeningitis serum was available anywhere in the city.[18] The laboratories of H. K. Mulford and Parke-Davis and Company simply could not keep up with the demand for their antimeningitis serum. Of note, Kansas City was not the only city requesting the serum from these companies. Desperate to obtain the serum, Dr. Wheeler finally appealed to the New York City Board of Health, which obliged "promptly and graciously" by sending a minimum of thirty doses per day of antimeningitis serum to Kansas City at an average cost of one dollar per dose. Dr. Park, ever vigilant about his budget, pointed out that even at this price, the New York City Board of Health was losing sixty cents per dose.[18] It is unknown why Dr. Wheeler and other physicians in Kansas City did not earlier request antimeningitis serum from the New York City Board of Health.

Without any antimeningitis serum with which to treat their patients for days in late March and early April 1912, the physicians at the Kansas City General Hospital administered intraspinal normal horse serum, normal salt solution, or phenol solution. One intern, Dr. Parmelee, reported, "These substitutes seemed to have [had] no influence on the disease. Improvement was seen in some from relief of pressure by withdrawal of spinal fluid but was only temporary. The patients thus treated either died or had a very protracted course."[28] Dr. Parmelee lamented that the situation had become so desperate that patients died who might have been saved could they have received the serum in time.[28]

Meanwhile, the weather during the final week of March 1912 remained cold and unstable. On Saturday, March 23, 1912, a snowstorm struck central and eastern Kansas that was the heaviest ever recorded in Kansas in the month of March. Topeka, about sixty miles west of Kansas City, received more than twelve inches of snow during the storm.[29] The precipitation shifted to rain on Saturday and Sunday, March 30 and 31, 1912, but temperatures dropped to freezing at night.[30]

CHAPTER 4 NOTES

1. William Lucien Gist, "Report on Meningitis," Hospital and Health Board, *Fourth Annual Report of the Hospital and Health Board of Kansas City, Missouri, for Fiscal Year April 17, 1911, to April 15, 1912, Inclusive* (Kansas City, MO: Hospital and Health Board, 1912), 55.

2. "Don't Be Afraid of Meningitis; That Is Don't Go Around Entertaining a Fear That You Will Get It; How to Avoid It; Pay Envelopes of Big Concerns in the Two Cities Last Week Contained Warning and Advice as to Nature and Spread of Disease," *Weekly Gazette Globe* (Kansas City, KS), March 7, 1912, 1.

3. "Mr. Hedrick Receiving Callers," *Kansas City Star*, March 1, 1912, 3.

4. "Fresh Air Best Antidote," *Kansas City Star*, March 3, 1912, 3.

5. Marie Ennis (1902–1912) was the only child of John William Ennis (1870–1960), the foreman of a wholesale produce company, and Leonora Ann Ennis (1875–1961).

6. "Four New Meningitis Cases; Three of Those Are Taken to the Hospital Today Are Negroes," *Kansas City Star*, March 4, 1912, 1. Note that the three other cases mentioned in this article were from Kansas City, Wyandotte County, Kansas.

7. "Marie Ennis," Missouri State Board of Health Bureau of Vital Statistics Certificate of Death, Registration District 899, File No. 9332, Primary Registration District No. 1002, and Registered No. 830.

8. "Three New Meningitis Cases; Marie Ennis, 10 Years Old, Died of the Disease Last Night," *Kansas City Star*, March 6, 1912, 3.

9. Dr. John Wesley Nixon (1871–1936) was born in Illinois as one of the six children of John Nixon (1822–1905) and Martha Ramsey (1837–1921). He earned his medical degree from the Marion Sims College of Medicine in St. Louis, Missouri, in 1896. He practiced medicine in Soldier, Jackson County, Kansas, for five years before moving to Kansas City, where he practiced medicine for thirty years in the same suite of offices in the Shukert Building on Grand Avenue. He married Eulah Porter (born in 1895) in 1922; they had no children. "Dr. John Wesley Nixon Dies; Physician Had Gone to Excelsior Springs to Recuperate," *Kansas City Star*, June 14, 1936, 4.

10. "Four New Meningitis Cases; Three of the Victims Reported Today Were Children," *Kansas City Star*, March 7, 1912, 6.

11. The Reverend Dr. Alexander Lewis (1864–1912) was born in Hudson, St. Croix County, Wisconsin. He earned his bachelor's degree from Carleton College in Northfield, Rice County, Minnesota, in 1887 and his divinity degree from Union Theological Seminary in New York in 1890. He earned his doctorate from New York University in 1892 and his doctor of divinity from Drury College in 1907. He married Ella Louisa Hatch (1862–1949) in 1890 and the same year was ordained to the ministry, becoming assistant pastor of Pilgrim Church, New York. Later, he was called to Pilgrim Church, Worcester, Massachusetts, and at the close of that pastorate, he spent a year abroad, studying at Oxford. While in England, he was a correspondent for the *Advance*, an evangelical newspaper. Upon his return to the United States, he was installed as the pastor of the First Church in Kansas City on October 25, 1906. He organized the work of the planning of the splendid building of the First Congregational Church, which he dreamed one day would become the cathedral of his denomination for the whole Midwest. "Rev. Alexander Lewis, D. D., '87," *Alumni Magazine, Carleton College, Northfield, Minnesota* 3, no.1 (May 1912), 17–21; and "Alexander Lewis," *Kansas City Star*, March 7, 1912, 8.

12. "Death Quick to Dr. Lewis; the Most Malignant Form of Spinal Meningitis; A Cold One Evening Developed Rapidly and Unconsciousness Came at 4 O'clock the Next Morning; Cases Widely Scattered," *Kansas City Star*, March 7, 1912, 2.

13. Dr. William Clay Morris (1852–1928) was born in Missouri as one of the three children of Dr. Joel T. Morris (1822–1872) and Margaret J. Simpson (1822–1904). He earned his medical degree from the College of Physicians and Surgeons of Kansas City in 1875. He married Inez Church (1855–1917) in 1882; they had no children. He died of a perforated ulcer. See "William Clay Morris," in Arthur Wayne Hafner, *Directory of Deceased American Physicians, 1804–1929* (Chicago, IL: American Medical Association, c. 1993).

14. Dr. Robert Tarleton Sloan (1861–1930) was born in Harrisonville, Cass County, Missouri, as one of the five children of Dr. Alfred Baxter Sloan (1827–1900) and Mary Ann Railey (1838–1887). In 1866, he moved with his family to Kansas City, where he graduated from Central High School in 1878. He earned his bachelor of arts and master of arts degrees from Missouri State University (Springfield, Greene County, Missouri) in 1883 and 1887, respectively, and his medical degree from the Medical Department of the University of

the City of New York in 1885. He returned to Kansas City, worked as the city chemist (1885–1886), and took over his father's Kansas City medical practice upon the latter's retirement. He served as the dean and professor of medicine at the Kansas City Medical College until it became a part of the University of Kansas School of Medicine in 1905. He lectured for ten years on heart and lung disease at the University of Kansas School of Medicine. He served as a president of the Jackson County Medical Society. He married Carrie Roberta Parks (1862–1930) in 1887; they had three children. He died at Research Hospital following an operation performed the previous week. He was sixty-nine years old. See *New York University Alumni Catalogue, 1833–1907, Medical Alumni: University Medical-Bellevue Hospital Medical-University and Bellevue Hospital Medical* (New York: General Alumni Society, 1908), 363; "Dr. Robert Sloan Dies; End Comes to a Long Career of Widely Known Physician; As a General Practitioner, Obstetrician, and Specialist in Internal Medicine; He Served Many Families Here," *Kansas City Star*, October 22, 1930, 10; and "Dr. Robert Tarlton [*sic*] Sloan," *Kansas City Medical Index-Lancet* 26, no. 2 (February 1905): 63.

15. "The Rev. Alexander Lewis," *Brooklyn Daily Eagle*, March 8, 1912, 3; "Rev. Alexander Lewis," *Tennessean* (Nashville, TN), March 8, 1912, 12; "Rev. Alexander Lewis Dies; Stricken with Meningitis—Was Ill Only Thirty Hours," *Sun* (New York, NY), March 8, 1912, 9; "Preacher Stricken with Meningitis," *Times-Democrat* (New Orleans, LA), March 8, 1912, 7; "Pastor Dies of Meningitis; Dr. Lewis of Kansas City One of Eight Victims; Eleven New Cases of the Malady Are Reported—Health Commissioner Says a Few Days of Sunshine Would Contribute Much to the Eradication of the Disease," *Los Angeles Times* (Los Angeles, CA), March 8, 1912, 5; "8 More Die of Meningitis; Eleven New Cases Reported at Kansas City—Officials Cannot Stop Spread of the Disease," *Brazil Daily Times* (Brazil, IN), March 8, 1912, 1.

16. "Four New Meningitis Cases; Three of the Victims Reported Today Were Children," *Kansas City Star*, March 7, 1912, 6.

17. "Pastor Dies of Meningitis; Dr. Lewis of Kansas City One of Eight Victims; Eleven New Cases of the Malady Are Reported—Health Commissioner Says a Few Days of Sunshine Would Contribute Much to the Eradication of the Disease," *Los Angeles Times*, March 8, 1912, 5.

18. "Treatment," Hospital and Health Board, *Fourth Annual Report of the Hospital and Health Board of Kansas City, Missouri, for Fiscal Year April 17, 1911, to April 15, 1912, Inclusive* (Kansas City, MO: Hospital and Health Board, 1912), 107.

19. "Don't Stay in the House! Get Out, Breathe the Air, and Exercise, a Doctor Advises," *Kansas City Star*, March 11, 1912, 1.

20. "Death of Mrs. L. I. Duncan; the Wife of the Council Sergeant-at-Arms Died of Meningitis," *Kansas City Star*, March 22, 1912, 2.

21. "Brief Bits of News," *Kansas City Star*, March 23, 1912, 8.

22. "Mrs. Mary C. Stafford Dead," *Kansas City Star*, March 24, 1912, 6.

23. "Death of Mrs. Emma Sisson," *Kansas City Star*, March 25, 1912, 2.

24. "Death of Miss Katherine Wolfe," *Kansas City Star*, April 1, 1912, 12.

25. Hospital and Health Board, "Contagious and Infectious Diseases Reported," *Monthly Report Hospital and Health Board, Kansas City, Missouri* 6, no. 3 (March 1912).

26. Hospital and Health Board, "Contagious Disease Cases Reported for the Year 1911–1912," *Fourth Annual Report of the Hospital and Health Board of Kansas City, Missouri, for Fiscal Year April 17, 1911, to April 15, 1912, Inclusive* (Kansas City, MO: Hospital and Health Board, 1912), 150.

27. In addition to the 113 case reports of cerebrospinal meningitis in Kansas City in March 1912, there were the following counts of other contagious diseases for the same month: diphtheria (seventeen cases) scarlet fever (forty-three), measles (twenty), chickenpox (thirty-nine), pneumonia (ninety-three), whooping cough (fifteen), mumps (eighteen), smallpox (three), typhoid fever (seven), and tuberculosis (twenty-one). For the second month in a row (February and March 1912), cerebrospinal meningitis was the leading cause of contagious-disease cases in Kansas City. Hospital and Health Board, "Contagious Disease Cases Reported for the Year 1911–1912," *Fourth Annual Report of the Hospital and Health Board of Kansas City, Missouri, for Fiscal Year April 17, 1911, to April 15, 1912, Inclusive* (Kansas City, MO: Hospital and Health Board, 1912), 150.

28. Arthur H. Parmelee, "Epidemic Cerebrospinal Meningitis," *Journal of the American Medical Association* 60, no. 9 (March 1, 1913): 660.

29. "The Snow Record in Kansas; Topeka Reports Snow the Depth in Various Parts of the State," *Kansas City Star*, March 25, 1912, 1.

30. "The Weather," *Kansas City Star*, March 30, 1912, 8.

CHAPTER 5

A FLOOD OF MIGHTY
WATERS, APRIL–JULY 1912

D uring the first days of April 1912, the snow blanketing
Kansas City finally turned to slush, the slush turned to
water, and antimeningitis serum flowed from the New
York City Board of Health to the Kansas City physicians caring
for cerebrospinal meningitis patients. Even with spring in the air,
Kansas City health department officials and private physicians
struggled to contain the exploding cerebrospinal meningitis
epidemic. During the first week of April 1912, there were twenty-
four new cases of cerebrospinal meningitis and twenty-six deaths
from it.[1] During the second week of April, there were thirty-one
new cases and thirty deaths.[2]

Around Tuesday, April 9, 1912, William Perry Motley, the
president of the Hospital and Health Board since 1909, contacted
Dr. Sophian in New York City to request his in-person help.[3–4]
It is unknown how Mr. Motley chose Dr. Sophian, although Dr.
Hall may have recommended him. The *Kansas City Post* (not the
Kansas City Star) underwrote the cost of Dr. Sophian's trip.[6] Dr.
Sophian had been planning to leave New York City on Monday,
April 22, 1912, to perform additional work in Dallas but agreed to
leave a week earlier to stop in Kansas City.[7] His wife, Estelle Felix
Sophian,[8] planned to accompany him on the trip.[9]

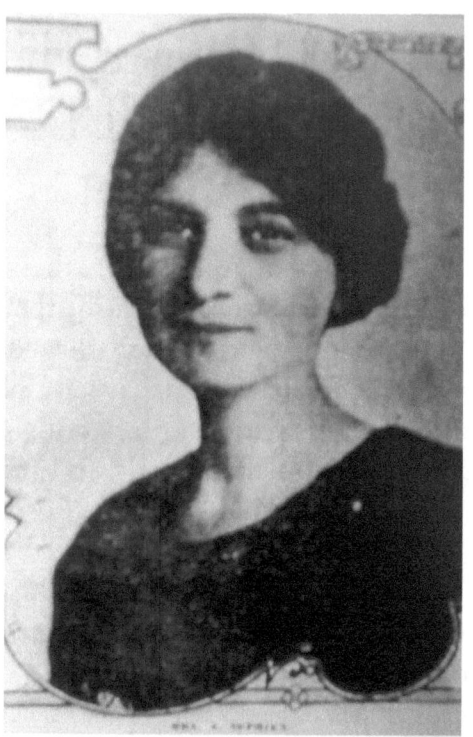

Estelle Felix Sophian (misspelled Sophien in caption) (1882–
1972), April 1912. Scanned from the *Kansas City Post*,
April 16, 1912, p. 1. The photographer is unknown.

Around Thursday, April 11, 1912, Dr. Sophian wired Mr. Motley: "Leaving New York Saturday, via St. Louis, arriving Kansas City 7:45 AM Monday morning. Have you enough serum? A. Sophian." Mr. Motley replied that he was glad to have him come, Kansas City had plenty of serum now, and he probably would have no trouble getting more.[4] The board expressed its commitment to Dr. Sophian to "use every possible means to block infection."[3]

Dr. Hasbrouck DeLamater,[10] an assistant health commissioner, and a representative of the *Kansas City Post* met Dr. and Mrs. Sophian at the Kansas City Depot at seven forty-five on the morning of Monday, April 15, 1912, and accompanied them to the Baltimore Hotel. Dr. Sophian rested for one hour before joining the members of the Hospital and Health Board to make plans to control the epidemic. The board provided to Dr. Sophian all possible information concerning the spread of cerebrospinal meningitis and the city's fruitless efforts to stamp it out. In addition, Dr. Sophian answered questions from board members concerning the epidemic. He remarked,

> Conditions here resemble those at Dallas, where I did special work last winter. There they had five cases in October, about fifty in December and two hundred in January. We plunged in and by scientific treatment of conditions in general checked the spread of the disease until it almost disappeared. I hope that we can do the same here in a few days, but I will remain here as long as it seems necessary. Just what steps will be taken first depends upon what I find in my investigations. I am surprised to learn this city has had so many cases.[7]

On Tuesday, April 16, 1912, word arrived in Kansas City that the RMS *Titanic*, the British passenger liner, had sunk in the North Atlantic Ocean. Dr. Sophian heard about the tragedy while paying a visit to the office of the *Kansas City Post*.[11] He spent the rest of the day with Dr. Wheeler and Dr. DeLamater, visiting every known cerebrospinal meningitis patient in Kansas City,[12] including the twenty-seven afflicted patients in the Kansas City General Hospital meningitis ward.[13] He gave lectures on cerebrospinal meningitis to the Hospital and Health Board, the Jackson County Medical Society, and the Wyandotte County Medical Society in Kansas.[14]

In his talk to the Wyandotte County Medical Society, Dr. Sophian noted that the meningococcus was of "very low" vitality and of short life and that under the most favorable circumstances in incubator cultures, it could not be kept alive more than three days without transplanting. The low vitality of the meningococcus prevented whole communities from being wiped out by it. Epidemics of the disease nearly always followed unusual climatic conditions, such as the Midwest had experienced in 1911–1912—that is, extremely hot and dry summer weather followed by unusually cold weather. He ventured that the manner by which these conditions triggered the epidemic was probably by a general lowering of the vitality of the people, thereby making them easy victims of the ravages of the meningitis germ.[14]

Dr. Sophian continued, saying that for every person infected by cerebrospinal meningitis, there were probably ten or more healthy carriers of the disease. A person could contract the disease from a healthy carrier just as easily as from a patient sick with the disease. He advised use of an antiseptic douche applied to the nasal cavities and a small dose of urotropin taken by mouth two or three times daily to reduce the number of healthy carriers of the meningococcus.[14]

How did one stop the spread of cerebrospinal meningitis in Kansas City? Dr. Sophian answered that there were only two ways: quarantine and vaccination. He believed that quarantining healthy carriers was impossible in a city as large as Kansas City. Recall that the Dallas approach to quarantine was to swab the nasal and throat passages of the contacts of afflicted individuals, culture the material from the swabs, identify the carriers of the meningococcus, quarantine the carriers, treat the carriers with antiseptic nasal and throat washes until their nose and throat cultures turned negative for the meningococcus, and then lift their quarantine.

Vaccination, the second way of stemming a cerebrospinal meningitis epidemic, was also difficult because people shied away from vaccinations. Dr. Sophian said, "It is very hard, at present, to convince anyone he should be given a meningitis vaccination to safeguard against the disease. Without these precautions, an epidemic of meningitis will continue indefinitely, except for when climatic conditions are such that it will die out of itself. Just what these conditions are is not known." He continued, "Vaccination has been a great success in Texas. Of the 185 persons to whom I administered vaccine myself, only one developed meningitis. This was a man who developed the disease three days after being given the vaccine, so there was no time for [the vaccine] to immunize."[15]

Dr. Sophian added, "The first symptoms of meningitis are like those of la grippe [flu]. They are a tired feeling, headache, dilated pupils of the eye, tenderness of skull and jaw, an irritable disposition, and slight fever. Persons suffering from ailments of this kind should not let them continue but should consult a physician and determine whether they have the first stage of the disease. Those who are given the serum during this stage recover, many of them in a few days."[15]

Then Dr. Sophian declared, "I believe that the epidemic in the two Kansas Citys and the Texas epidemic were caused by the same source. What that source is has not been determined. The high death rate here is due to the fact that few cases are treated in early stages of the disease."[15] Dr. Sophian ended his speech by saying that a few weeks of mild weather and proper care by all the people in Kansas City would probably wipe out the disease.[14]

If someone in Kansas City decided to undertake a vaccination program there, where would he obtain the meningococcal vaccine? There were at least two sources of heat-killed meningococcal vaccine. Dr. VanAtta was manufacturing a heat-killed meningococcal vaccine in the pathology laboratory of the Kansas City General Hospital for use in an unknown number of willing hospital staff, as noted above.[16] It was unlikely he would or could manufacture sufficient meningococcal vaccine to inoculate the large number of people who would qualify to receive it—that is, those people exposed to an individual with the disease.

The second source of meningococcal vaccine was the H. K. Mulford Company, which, in April 1912, released Meningo-Bacterin, the first commercially produced heat-killed meningococcal vaccine. The company noted that its meningococcal vaccine had "thus far been used in relatively few cases, yet it was entirely reasonable to believe that it will prove a most valuable aid in the suppression of epidemics of cerebrospinal meningitis."[17] In its advertisement for Meningo-Bacterin in the *Medical Herald* in April 1912, the H. K. Mulford Company shared its method of preparing its meningococcal vaccine,[18] provided directions on how to administer the vaccine,[19] and outlined how it supplied the vaccine for use by physicians.[20]

Dr. Frank Hall stepped forward to orchestrate a meningococcal vaccination program in April 1912 to prevent cerebrospinal meningitis in individuals exposed to patients with the disease. He vaccinated fifty exposed families (around 280 people in all) and a number of physicians, nurses, and other hospital staff. He apparently gave each person the full three doses. No one developed appreciable side effects from the vaccine, and no one who had received the vaccine subsequently developed cerebrospinal meningitis. Dr. Hall's undertaking currently is known to history through its mention in a national speech by Dr. Sophian and in two of Dr. Sophian's writings.[21–22]

What did Dr. Gist, Dr. Luscher, and Dr. Wheeler think about a meningococcal vaccine? Dr. Gist joined Dr. Hall as a strong advocate of the vaccine to prevent cerebrospinal meningitis. In April 1912, after meeting Dr. Sophian in Kansas City, Dr. Gist said,

> The prevention of the development of cerebrospinal meningitis is our strongest achievement. It has been proven beyond a doubt that the meningococci vaccine is of excellent service. An immunity of the

second or third order is developed in the body by its use (Sophian) [sic]. By its discreet and liberal use in an epidemic, it is my belief the disease can be stamped out. It is the best practical solution of rational prophylaxis. This disease should be handled as we do smallpox, i.e., isolation of cases, vaccination of exposed people, quarantining of premises and fumigation.[23]

Dr. Luscher also championed a meningococcal vaccine after Dr. Sophian's visit to Kansas City, writing, "A preventive in the form of vaccination has been found. The idea has been experimented with some time, but since the recent epidemic in Texas and here, vaccination has been proved an absolute safeguard. Anyone fearing meningitis should be vaccinated."[24]

Dr. Wheeler was more circumspect about the value of a meningococcal vaccine after Dr. Sophian's visit to Kansas City. He never could bring himself to use the term *meningococcal vaccine* in his writings and insisted that the most important requirements (in order of most to least important) to stem a cerebrospinal meningitis epidemic were to secure "earnest cooperation between the people and the health authorities in the enforcing of all necessary health regulations," quarantine all people stricken with the disease, cleanse all tenement houses and prevent "large numbers of the lower classes of our citizenship packing together in poorly ventilated hovels," render "healthy germ carriers harmless," use "all possible force in the power of health authorities to cause all cases to be treated in hospitals," and practice good oral and nasal hygiene.[25] He added, "Quarantine measures, however strict, to check the spread of this disease are not only absurd but unscientific."[26]

It is plausible that Dr. Sophian visited Dr. Hall's American Biologic Company during his visit to Kansas City in April 1912. The laboratory was located on the seventh floor of the Gloyd Building at 921 Walnut Street. Dr. Hall likely told Dr. Sophian about the recent departure of his longtime laboratory director, a homeopathic physician who had returned to Pennsylvania to direct a major laboratory there.[27] Dr. Hall also likely expressed concern about the difficulty of obtaining adequate supplies of sera and vaccines in Kansas City. It is probable that Dr. Hall said that Kansas City could benefit from a local biologics company established and operated by people of the caliber of those working at the Research Laboratory of the New York City Board of Health. What did Dr. Sophian think about this idea?[28]

Dr. Wheeler was grateful to Dr. Sophian for visiting Kansas City, writing,

> It is somewhat satisfying to mention that our work received the strong endorsement of the distinguished specialist, Dr. Sophian, of New York City, who so successfully conducted the epidemic in Dallas, Texas ... You recall that Dr. Sophian addressed this Board upon the subject of Cerebro-Spinal Meningitis and told us that he had nothing to add to what was already carried out by your Health Commissioner and the staff of physicians in the General Hospital. He did, however, suggest one point which I adopted at once, namely, that the serum to be used in the treatment of this disease should be entirely controlled by the Hospital and Health Board.[6, 29]

Dr. and Mrs. Sophian departed Kansas City for Dallas, Texas, by train late Thursday, April 18, 1912, and arrived at the latter city on Friday night, April 19, 1912. As they registered at the Park Hotel, Dr. Sophian told reporters, "My visit to Dallas has no connection with existing conditions. [The city remained in the throes of its cerebrospinal meningitis epidemic.] I wish that to be clearly understood, because the disease was practically stamped out here some time ago [when Dr. Sophian left Dallas in early February 1912]. My object in coming to Dallas at this time is simply to complete some studies which I did not have time to finish during my stay here in the winter." Dr. Sophian continued, "In these experiments Dr. [James Harvey] Black[30] will assist me in the laboratory of the Southwestern Medical College. Our object will be to ascertain just how much protection vaccination affords against attacks of meningitis. We hope to be able to work out something that will be of value in handling future epidemics of meningitic. I do not know just how long these studies will engage us, but we shall prosecute them for several weeks at all events."[31]

When asked about his experience in Kansas City, Dr. Sophian replied, "The epidemic at Kansas City, which was about as violent as that in Dallas, has very much abated. The local Health Board adopted practically the same measures that were employed in Dallas, and I am very much pleased with the results. The situation there is well under control."[31]

Why did Dr. Sophian return to Dallas to perform research on the meningococcal vaccine, when Dr. Thayer had been doing so? The reason was that on Sunday, February 18, 1912, Dr. Thayer had resigned from his pathology professorship at the Baylor University College of Medicine in Dallas to become the medical supervisor of the Texas Baptist Memorial Hospital in Dallas.[32] He had ended his meningococcal vaccine studies and closed his laboratory. He did publish a summary of his meningococcal vaccine work in the *Texas State Journal of Medicine* in March 1912.[33]

A description of the innovative research on the efficacy and safety of the meningococcal vaccine performed by Dr. Sophian and Dr. Black in Texas is available elsewhere.[34] In brief, they provided evidence to support the efficacy of the heat-killed meningococcal vaccine in preventing cerebrospinal meningitis for up to two years after a person's initial vaccination.[35] Dr. and Mrs. Sophian returned to New York City on Friday, May 10, 1912.

Meanwhile, back in Kansas City, the Hospital and Health Board counted eighty-two cases of cerebrospinal meningitis for the month of April 1912; it continued to be most prevalent contagious disease in Kansas City for that month.[36] The total case count for cerebrospinal meningitis in Kansas City between January 1, 1912, and April 30, 1912, was 280, according to the Hospital and Health Board data. The prevalence of cerebrospinal meningitis in Kansas

City between January 1, 1912, and April 30, 1912, according to the data collected by the Hospital and Health Board, calculated to *11.2 cerebrospinal meningitis cases per 10,000 Kansas City residents.*

The weather in early May 1912 in Kansas City was generally fair and warm, with high temperatures in the midseventies and mideighties and low temperatures in the midsixties.[37] Basking in the balmy May weather, Dr. DeLamater declared, "The epidemic of cerebrospinal meningitis in Kansas City is over." He added, "The change to warm weather and the general cleanup of the city within the last few weeks have produced that result. The epidemic has been on the decline and within the danger line for a month. We have had no deaths and no new cases for two days and the number of patients in the isolation ward at the General Hospital has very much decreased." He concluded, "It is my opinion that there need be no further fear from the disease."[38]

The number of new cerebrospinal meningitis cases reported to the Hospital and Health Board for May 1912 plummeted to fourteen (down from eighty-two in April 1912), with thirty deaths.[39] In June 1912, the number of new cases of cerebrospinal meningitis reported to the Hospital and Health Board was fifteen, with nine deaths. In July 1912, the Hospital and Health Board received reports of seven new cases of cerebrospinal meningitis and seven deaths from the disease.[40]

Around Saturday, June 1, 1912, Dr. Wheeler, Dr. Gist, Dr. Luscher, Dr. Pipkin, and Dr. Parmelee provided independent accounts of the cerebrospinal meningitis epidemic of Kansas City during the fiscal year from mid-April 1911 to mid-April 1912. Dr. Wheeler wrote,

> I have the honor to submit herewith my report upon the development, extent and result of the recent epidemic of cerebrospinal meningitis. The tables and figures in this report are based upon 414 cases that were reported to the Department of Health from January 1st to June 1st, 1912 ...

Based on a population of 300,000, the prevalence of cerebrospinal meningitis in this epidemic was quite marked, *13.8 cases per 10,000*. [When the truer population of 250,000 is used to calculate prevalence, the rate becomes *16.6 cerebrospinal meningitis cases per 10,000 Kansas City residents* from January 1, 1912, to June 1, 1912.] This is slightly in excess of many epidemics in the United States. In New York in the year 1872 the rate was 8.07 cases per 10,000 [here, Dr. Wheeler mistook the New York City cerebrospinal meningitis mortality rate for the disease's prevalence rate]. In 1905 it was 6.30 cases per 10,000 [again, Dr. Wheeler mistook the New York City mortality rate for the prevalence rate]; Glasgow, in 1907, it was 8.47 cases per 1,000; Paris, in 1909, it was less than 1 case per 10,000.[40]

Dr. Wheeler's sum of 414 cases of cerebrospinal meningitis during the Kansas City epidemic, January 1, 1912, to June 1, 1912, suggests that between May 1, 1912, and June 1, 1912, the board had counted 134 additional cases. Recall that the Hospital and Health Board had counted 280 cases of the disease at the end of April 30, 1912.

Dr. Gist wrote,

The rate of mortality in this epidemic was unusually high for cases treated with serum. The average mortality rate of cases treated without serum is 70 to 85 percent. In Flexner's series of 712 cases (collective) treated with his serum prepared by himself, the mortality rate was 31.4. These cases were collected in about the same manner as ours which included the moribund cases as they entered the hospitals or were treated privately at home. Our mortality rate was 53.55 plus, the excessiveness of which I am unable to explain, except it be an unmatured quality of serum due to the excessive demand upon the producers. The serum of the New York Board of Health proved therapeutically to be a marked improvement over that furnished by other biological houses.[41]

Dr. Luscher wrote,

Cerebrospinal Meningitis [sic] prevailed in our community in epidemic form, beginning in December 1911. To the end of the fiscal year, April 15, 1912, there were treated here [Kansas City General Hospital] 216 cases. Twenty-nine cases remaining in the hospital. [sic] While the epidemic appears to be abating, new cases are frequent. Right here I wish to report to you that our resident staff of physicians (interns), nurses, and other attendants deserve special commendation for their bravery and devotion, when people throughout the city and country were in a state of panic from fear. The mortality was frightful. Of those brought to General Hospital, 52.6 percent died. However, deducting those who died within the first 24 hours, practically moribund when they came to us, 42.5 percent died. When we deduct all those over 50 years of age, who invariably died, and those under 2 years of age, of whom 64 percent died, we find a comparatively low mortality for this disease of 41.7 percent.[42]

Dr. Pipkin wrote that forty-six African Americans had been treated for cerebrospinal meningitis at the Old Hospital between January 1, 1912, and June 1, 1912. Dr. Pipkin added, "It was several weeks after the appearance of cerebrospinal meningitis in this city that any negroes contracted this disease. Our high death rate, 69.3 percent, is due in a measure to their late arrival at the hospital, consequently the late use of the serum. The cases received and treated since the close of the fiscal year do not appreciably lower the death rate."[43]

Dr. Parmelee published in the *Journal of the American Medical Association* the data and experience of the physician team caring for the cerebrospinal meningitis patients admitted to Kansas City General Hospital between January 1, 1912, and June 1, 1912. As of June 1, 1912, the team had cared for 230 patients, of whom 121 had died (a 53 percent mortality rate), 108 had recovered, and one was still convalescing. Dr. Parmelee reported a mortality rate of 52.6 percent and provided a number of remarks he thought would be of interest to readers. For example, he noted that the average duration of illness of the cerebrospinal meningitis patients admitted to the Kansas City General Hospital was 12.8 days.[44] He also noted,

> The method of administering serum was practically the same in all cases, modified of course by the age and general condition of the patient. An initial dose of from 30 to 55 c.c. [*sic*] was usually give to adult patients as soon as they reached the hospital; a second injection of from 20 to 30 c.c. was given from 12 to 18 hours later; and subsequently one or two doses of from 20 to 30 c.c. and a dose or two of from ten to fifteen cubic centimeters at intervals of twenty-four hours. The continuance of the serum treatment depended, of course, on whether or not meningococci were still present in the spinal fluid.[44]

Dr. Parmelee also wrote,

> Epidemics differ so in their severity that it is not possible to state to what extent the serum treatment influenced the mortality in this epidemic. Nevertheless, I am convinced, first, that the course of the disease was materially shortened in those cases that showed any response to treatment [with

antimeningitis serum]; second, that complications and sequelae were much less frequent, and third, that the remarkable results obtained in many cases seen early in the course of the disease were due to the specific action of the serum on the infection.[45]

On Thursday, July 18, 1912, Dr. Luscher discharged the last cerebrospinal meningitis patient from the Kansas City General Hospital, fumigated and disinfected the meningitis ward, and returned it to service as a general medical ward. Dr. Luscher advised people who feared contracting cerebrospinal meningitis to receive the meningococcal vaccination, as noted earlier.[24] Dr. Luscher's final words to the public on the cerebrospinal meningitis epidemic in 1912 were,

> There is no more danger to be looked for from meningitis in Kansas City this summer. It is probable that a few sporadic cases will become evident, but that always has been the history of the disease. We are hoping to safeguard against a general epidemic [in 1912–1913] as we have experienced this fall [1911] and winter [1912]. The history of the disease indicates that there will be a return of it this fall [1912]. It may be light or it may be heavy. We hope that it will not reappear, but of several previous epidemics, the facts show that the disease usually has returned and sometimes with renewed vigor.[24]

On Saturday, July 27, 1912, the new contagious-diseases hospital building was complete. However, the city government lacked the $4,000 to furnish it, so it sat empty.[46]

CHAPTER 5 NOTES

1. "Cerebrospinal Meningitis: Cases and Deaths Reported by City Health Authorities for the Week Ended April 6, 1912," *Public Health Reports* 27, no. 18 (May 3, 1912): 619.

2. "Cerebrospinal Meningitis: Cases and Deaths Reported by City Health Authorities for the Week Ended April 13, 1912," *Public Health Reports* 27, no. 17 (April 26, 1912): 651.

3. "Sophian Going to Kansas City; Spinal Meningitis Expert Will Aid in Stamping Out Disease in That City," *Dallas Morning News*, April 11, 1912, 7.

4. "NY Meningitis Expert Will Be in KC Monday; Dr. A. Sophien [*sic*] Wires Perry H. Motley, of Hospital and Health Board, He Will Start Saturday; Disease Claims 4 More Victims; Two New Cases Reported; City Now Well Supplied with Serum and Another Famine Not Likely," *Kansas City Post*, April 11, 1912, 1.

5. The *Kansas City Post* was a large newspaper in Kansas City from 1854 to 1942. See "From Local Project to Lively Pioneer: A Short History of the *Kansas City Journal-Post*," University of Missouri at Kansas City, accessed May 14, 2018, https://web.archive.org/web/20071212012313/http://library.umkc.edu/spec-col/journalpost/jp-intro.htm.

6. "Cerebro-Spinal Meningitis, Report on Meningitis," Hospital and Health Board, *Fourth Annual Report of the Hospital and Health Board of Kansas City, Missouri, for Fiscal Year April 17, 1911, to April 15, 1912, Inclusive* (Kansas City, MO: Hospital and Health Board, 1912), 55.

7. "Meningitis Expert Arrives in KC to Combat Disease; Dr. A. Sophien [*sic*], World Famous Specialist, Surprised at Extent of Its Ravages; Consults Local Men; Says He Will Remain Here as Long as Is Necessary to Check Spread," *Kansas City Post*, April 15, 1912, 1; and "Dr. Sophian to Fight Disease; Meningitis Expert Says Conditions in Kansas City Resemble Those at Dallas Last Winter," *Dallas Morning News*, April 16, 1912, 11.

8. Estelle Felix Sophian (1882–1972) was born in Warta, Posen, Prussia, as the sixth of the eight children of Arthur A. Felix (1855–1930) and Emilie Leitner (1855–1912). The family immigrated in separate groups, with Arthur A., Sarah, Pauline, Eva, and Joseph arriving in Buffalo, Erie County, New York, in December 1890 and Emilie, Flora, Estelle, Louis, and Eugenia arriving in Buffalo in May 1891.

The family subsequently moved from Buffalo to New York City, where Estelle attended the Normal College of the City of New York for four years, graduating at the age of seventeen years in 1900. Estelle Felix earned the second-best academic record in her class (Agnes Peterson was number one by a hair) and had an almost perfect attendance record for four years. At the normal-course graduation, she won the William Wood Memorial Prize (forty dollars in gold) for making the greatest progress in French and received an honorable mention for the Wilson G. Hunt Gold Medal for Latin. If Estelle had studied at the school for one more year, she would have been eligible to receive a bachelor's degree. The Normal College of the City of New York offered a normal course of four years and an academic course of five years; the latter resulted in a bachelor of arts degree. The purpose of the normal course was to furnish New York City with a constant supply of trained teachers. After graduating from the Normal School, Estelle Felix taught primary school in the New York City public school system for at least a decade. Estelle's younger sister, Eugenie (Jane) Felix (1885–1945), married Harry Sophian (1882–1945) in 1907. Harry Sophian, a real estate agent and developer, was Dr. Abraham Sophian's older brother. Estelle Felix married Dr. Abraham Sophian on Wednesday, April 26, 1911, in New York City. See *Manual of the Normal College of the City of New York, 1894* (New York: Douglas Taylor and Company, 1894), 35–36; *Directory of Teachers in the Public Schools* (New York: Board of Education of the City of New York, 1905), 160; *Thirtieth Annual Report of the Normal College for the Year Ending December 31, 1900; Catalogue of the Students Together with the Class Standing of Each Student* (New York: Regents of the State of New York, 1900), 25, 51, 86; and "Normal College Graduates," *School* 11, no. 2 (September 19, 1899), 341. For images of the students and faculty of the Normal College in 1896 and 1897, see *Normal College Echo, First Annual, 1896* (New York: J. S. Babcock, 1896); and *Normal College Echo, Second Annual, 1897* (New York: J. S. Babcock, 1897).

9. "Dr. Sophien's [*sic*] Wife Finds Much Charm in Kansas City; Eminent Specialist's 'Better Half' Calls Trip Second Honeymoon; Faith in Mate Great; Expresses Pleasure with Bustle and Window Displays Here on First Visit West," *Kansas City Post*, April 17, 1912, 2.

10. Dr. Hasbrouck DeLamater (1870–1953) was born in Kingston, Ulster County, New York, as the son of Meluan DeLamater and Susan Jane Carney. His place of medical training is unknown. He

served seven years under Dr. Walter S. Wheeler as an assistant health commissioner of Kansas City, Missouri (1908–1915). He left Kansas City to become the health commissioner of St. Joseph, Buchanan County, Missouri, and medical director of that city's public schools. Dr. DeLamater married Harriet Rachael "Isabella" Taylor (1872–1965) in 1907; they had no children. He died at the age of eighty-three years after a long illness. "Delamater to St. Joseph; New City and School Health Director Was Official Here; Record in Kansas City Brought Indorsement of Federal Inspectors and Led to Appointment; Pays $3,600 a Year," *Kansas City Star*, December 14, 1916, 7; and "Former St. Joseph Health Director Dies," *Macon Chronicle* (Macon, MO), September 25, 1953, 1.

11. "Climate Declared to Be Responsible for Meningitis; Dr. A. Sophien [*sic*], New York Expert, Explains Cause, Preventive, and Cure; To Address Doctors; Situation Here Well Handled He Says—In KC to Aid Health Officials," *Kansas City Post*, April 16, 1912, 1.

12. Hospital and Health Board, "Medical Diseases—General Hospital, From April 16, 1912, to April 21, 1913," *Fifth Annual Report of the Hospital and Health Board of Kansas City, Missouri, for Fiscal Year April 16, 1912, to April 21, 1913, Inclusive* (Kansas City, MO: Hospital and Health Board, 1913), 135.

13. "No New Meningitis Cases; Apparently a Check in the Disease, Say Health Officers," *Kansas City Star*, April 15, 1912, 1.

14. "Meningitis Germ Is Explained; Specialist Tells the Nature of the Germ—When and How Disease Becomes Epidemic; Cold Weather Visitor; Health Persons May Carry It Around and Infect Others Whose Systems Are Susceptible—Epidemic Due to Weather Conditions," *Weekly Gazette Globe*, April 18, 1912, 1.

15. "Only 2 Ways to Stop Meningitis Spread, He Says; Dr. Sophian, New York Expert, Lectures Wyandotte County Medical Society; He May Leave Tonight; Specialist to Visit Children Impaired by Ravages of the Disease," *Kansas City Post*, April 18, 1912, 1.

16. Dr. VanAtta wrote around April 1912, "Stock typhoid and meningococcic vaccines are made in the laboratory and given to those in constant contact with these diseases." Hospital and Health Board, *Fourth Annual Report of the Hospital and Health Board of Kansas City, Missouri, for Fiscal Year April 17, 1911, to April 15, 1912, Inclusive* (Kansas City, MO: Hospital and Health Board, 1912): 28.

17. "Interesting Announcement Is Made in This Issue by the H. K. Mulford Company Concerning Meningo-Bacterin (Meningococcus Vaccine)," *Medical Herald* 31, no. 4 (April 1912): 205.

18. The H. K. Mulford Company made its meningococcal vaccine "by growing meningococci on a serum agar for about 24 hours, washing off the meningococci and suspending them in a salt solution, counting by Wright's method a set number of meningococci in one cubic centimeter of the suspension, and then killing the meningococci in the suspension by heating them to, say, 60 degrees Centigrade (140 degrees Fahrenheit) for a certain amount of time, say one-half hour or more. After dilution of the thick suspension with normal saline solution, so that different strengths of the vaccine could be obtained, the now-completed vaccine was tested aerobically and anaerobically to demonstrate the sterility of the vaccine (i.e., the absence of live meningococci or their spores). Additional tests in guinea pigs or other animals were conducted to rule out the existence of harmful substances in the vaccine. A preservative, such as Trikresol (0.25 percent), was added to the suspension as a preservative." "Interesting Announcement Is Made in This Issue by the H. K. Mulford Company Concerning Meningo-Bacterin (Meningococcus Vaccine)," *Medical Herald* 31, no. 4 (April 1912): 205.

19. The H. K. Mulford Company provided the following directions for administering Meningo-Bacterin: "The usual site for inoculation is the arm at about the insertion of the deltoid muscle. The dose is given subcutaneously and not into the muscle nor into the skin. An area about the size of a five-cent piece is painted with tincture of iodine. The syringe needle is plunged through this area. No after treatment is necessary. The complete immunization treatment consists of three doses given at intervals of from five to ten days. The first dose is 500 million [killed meningococci bacteria], the second dose 1000 million and the third dose 1000 million. For children smaller doses should be used according to weight. It has been suggested that the unit of body weight for a full dose be considered 150 pounds." "Interesting Announcement Is Made in This Issue by the H. K. Mulford Company Concerning Meningo-Bacterin (Meningococcus Vaccine)," *Medical Herald* 31, no. 4 (April 1912): 205.

20. The H. K. Mulford Company provided the following information on the packaging of the Meningo-Bacterin vaccine: "Meningo-Bacterin for Immunizing Is Supplied in Two Distinct Style of Packages: First. —For immunizing one person there are supplied three syringes, each

containing the proper amount for injection, designated respectively, first, second, and third doses. The first syringe contains the initial dose of 500 million killed minigococci [*sic*], and the second and third 1000 million each. The contents of the first syringe are to be followed five to ten days later by the contents of the second syringe and again five to ten days later by the contents of the third. Second. —For immunizing ten persons, meningo-bacterin is supplied in hospital or board of health packages containing 30 ampules or ten complete immunizing doses. The initial doses (500 million killed bacteria) are contained in the ampuls with the red label, the second doses (1000 million killed bacteria) in ampuls with the white label and the third dose (1000 killed bacteria) in ampuls with the blue label. In each case the first injection is 500 million (red label), the second 1000 million (white label), is administered five to ten days later, and the third of 1000 million (blue label) is injected five to ten days following the second injection. No syringe is supplied with the hospital size package, since it is expected that physicians using the same will employ their own hypodermic syringe, after sterilization. The method of withdrawing the vaccine from the ampul is to moisten the rubber top or cap with a drop of liquor cresolis comp., U. S. P. or 5 percent solution of carbolic acid; push the needle through the drop of antiseptic [*sic*] on the rubber cap, and then invert the bottle and slowly withdraw the required amount for injecting, following the instructions for the three injections necessary as directed. The H. K. Mulford Company also supply [*sic*] antimeningitis serum prepared after the method of Flexner and Jobling, and they will mail upon request to the Philadelphia office, Mulford Working Bulletin No. 8, on Anti-Meningitis Serum, giving a detailed and impartial review of the literature." "Interesting Announcement Is Made in This Issue by the H. K. Mulford Company Concerning Meningo-Bacterin (Meningococcus Vaccine)," *Medical Herald* 31, no. 4 (April 1912): 205–6.

21. Abraham Sophian and James Harvey Black, "Prophylactic Vaccination against Epidemic Meningitis," *Transactions of the Section on Pathology and Physiology of the American Medical Association at the Sixty-Third Annual Session, Held at Atlantic City, NJ, June 4 to 7, 1912* (Chicago, IL: American Medical Association, 1912): 59.

22. Abraham Sophian, *Epidemic Cerebrospinal Meningitis* (St. Louis, MO: C. V. Mosby, 1913), 197.

23. William Lucien Gist, Hospital and Health Board, *Fourth Annual Report of the Hospital and Health Board of Kansas City, Missouri, for Fiscal Year April 17, 1911, to April 15, 1912, Inclusive* (Kansas City, MO: Hospital and Health Board, 1912), 108.

24. "Last Stand of Meningitis; General Hospital Finally Free of Cases of the Disease; No More Danger of the Malady Need Be Looked for This Summer, Doctor Luscher Says, But a Return Scourge Is Probable the Coming Winter," *Kansas City Star*, July 18, 1912, 12.

25. "Report on Meningitis: Treatment," Hospital and Health Board, *Fourth Annual Report of the Hospital and Health Board of Kansas City, Missouri, for Fiscal Year April 17, 1911, to April 15, 1912, Inclusive* (Kansas City, MO: Hospital and Health Board, 1912), 107.

26. "Cerebro-Spinal Meningitis, Report on Meningitis," Hospital and Health Board, *Fourth Annual Report of the Hospital and Health Board of Kansas City, Missouri, for Fiscal Year April 17, 1911, to April 15, 1912, Inclusive* (Kansas City, MO: Hospital and Health Board, 1912), 57–58.

27. Dr. Hall's laboratory director from 1909 to 1912 was Dr. Edwin Lightner Nesbit (1878–1929), a homeopathic physician. Dr. Nesbit was born in Lewisburg, Union County, Pennsylvania, as the eldest of the four children of Joseph C. Nesbit (1848–1917), an architect and builder, and Rebecca M. Lightner (1855–1931). He received his early formal education in the Lewisburg public schools and at Bucknell Academy, earned his bachelor's degree from Bucknell University in 1899, and earned his homeopathic medical degree at Hahnemann Medical College of Philadelphia in 1904. From 1904 to 1909, he practiced medicine in Bryn Mawr, Delaware County, Pennsylvania. From 1909 to 1912, he directed Dr. Frank J. Hall's American Biologic Company in Kansas City. He then moved back to Philadelphia to direct the Constantine Hering Laboratory at the Hahnemann Medical College. In 1924, he moved to Florida, where he died in an automobile accident in 1929. He married Grace Maude Gore (1876–1965) in 1920. They had no children. See "Eleven Students Risk Lives for Study of Drug; Dr. Edwin L. Nesbit Makes Important Medical Tests; Important Experiments to Determine Caffeine's Effect Conducted at Hahnemann," *Philadelphia Inquirer*, May 12, 1912, 1.

28. Dr. Hall was given credit for persuading Dr. Sophian to move to Kansas City to establish a serum and vaccine laboratory and farm. See "Anti-Toxin Farm at Kansas City: Scientists Will Supply World

with Serum; Dr. Sophian of New York, Who Helped Stamp Out Meningitis There, One of the Members," *Chillicothe Morning Constitution* (Chillicothe, MO), August 5, 1912, 1.

29. "To Turn Over All Serum to Health Board; Physicians Must Get Medicine to Fight Meningitis From the General Hospital," *Kansas City Post*, April 17, 1912, 8.

30. Dr. James Harvey Black (1884–1958) was born in Huntington, Cabell County, West Virginia, as one of the six children of the Reverend James Adam Black (1854–1902) and Mary Nancy Murphy (1856–1942). James Harvey Black moved with his family to Fannin, Goliad County, Texas, in 1900; his father died two years later. James Harvey Black graduated from Paris (Texas) High School in 1900 and spent two years preparing for medical college at the Academic Department of Southwestern University in Georgetown, Williamson County, Texas. He then moved to Dallas, where he earned his medical degree from the Southwestern University Medical Department in 1907. Dr. Black served an internship at nearby St. Paul's Sanitarium (1906–1907), returned to 1420 Hall Street as a professor, and lectured medical students on bacteriology (1907–1911). In 1911, Southwestern University Medical Department became Southern Methodist University Medical Department, and Dr. Black became professor of bacteriology and pathology at the latter institution. He was also dean of Southern Methodist University Medical Department (1914–1915), when the trustees of Southern Methodist University closed the medical department and merged the school's assets with Baylor University College of Medicine. From 1915 to 1942, Dr. Black was professor of bacteriology and pathology, preventive medicine, and clinical medicine at the Baylor University College of Medicine. In 1942, he became a professor of clinical medicine at Southwestern Medical School, a new school. Dr. Black maintained a private practice in clinical pathology in the Wilson Building on Main Street in downtown Dallas (1907–1932). In 1932, he limited his practice to allergies. He married Allena Marie Patton (1886–1978) in 1913; they had two children. He died of a coronary occlusion at the age of seventy-four years. See *Sou'wester Yearbook 1907*, Southwestern University (Georgetown, Texas: Athletic Association of Southwestern University, 1907), 160–61; "Dr. J. H. Black Dies, SMS [*sic*] Allergy Specialist," *Dallas Morning News*, December 1, 1958, 5; "In Memoriam, James Harvey Black, 1884–1958," *American Journal of Clinical Pathology* 32, no. 2 (August

1959): 172–73; "On Trail of Hay Fever; Allergy Causes Are Elusive, Physician Concludes," *Kansas City Times*, September 21, 1950, 3; "SMU's Forgotten Medical School," *SMU Magazine*, accessed January 3, 2018, http://blog.smu.edu/smumagazine/2011/12/smus-forgotten-medical-school/; and "Banquet to Dr. J. H. Black; Southwestern Medical Dean Going to Kentucky to Wed," *Dallas Morning News*, August 20, 1913, 6.

31. "Will Complete Experiments; Dr. Sophian Returns to Study Value of Vaccination against Meningitis," *Dallas Morning News*, April 20, 1912, 9.

32. "To Improve Baptist Hospital: Plans Now Being Made for Closer Affiliation with Medical College; Supervisor Is Named," *Dallas Morning News*, February 18, 1912, 7; "Baylor University College of Medicine" (advertisement), *Dallas Morning News,* August 4, 1912, 13; and Walter Henrik Moursund, *A History of Baylor University, College of Medicine, 1900–1953* (Houston, TX: Gulf Printing Company, 1956), 37–50, 55–56.

33. Alfred Edward Thayer, "The Dallas Epidemic of Meningitis; Preliminary Note on the Laboratory Work," *Texas State Journal of Medicine* 7, no. 11 (March 1912): 305–7.

34. Drs. Sophian and Black inoculated ten volunteer medical students with the experimental meningococcal vaccine, studied the students' blood for the presence of immune bodies, and found those immune bodies, which provided evidence that the students had developed immunity to the meningococcus. Dr. Black restudied the medical students one year and two years after their initial immunizations, in 1913 and 1914, and found that they still had immunity to the meningococcus. Drs. Sophian and Black published their seminal paper on the meningococcal vaccine—"Prophylactic Vaccination against Epidemic Meningitis"—in *Journal of the American Medical Association* 59, no. 7 (August 17, 1912): 527–32.

35. Dr. Black published the one-year and two-year follow-up studies as James Harvey Black, "Prophylactic Vaccination against Epidemic Meningitis," *Journal of the American Medical Association* 60, no. 17 (April 26, 1913): 1289–90; and James Harvey Black, "Prophylactic Vaccination against Epidemic Meningitis, a Supplementary Note," *Journal of the American Medical Association* 68, no. 24 (December 12, 1914): 2126.

36. Hospital and Health Board, "Contagious and Infectious Diseases Reported," *Monthly Report of the Hospital and Health Board,*

Kansas City, Missouri 6, no. 4 (April 1912); and Hospital and Health Board, "Contagious Disease Cases Reported for the Year 1911–1912," *Fourth Annual Report of the Hospital and Health Board of Kansas City, Missouri, for Fiscal Year April 17, 1911, to April 15, 1912, Inclusive* (Kansas City, MO: Hospital and Health Board, 1912), 150.

37. "The Weather—Fair," *Kansas City Star*, May 1, 1912, 1; "The Weather—Showers, Cooler," *Kansas City Star*, May 2, 1912, 1; and "The Weather," *Kansas City Star*, May 3, 1912, 8.

38. "No Deaths and No New Cases Reported for Two Days and the Health Department Says There Should Be No Further Fear," *Kansas City Star*, May 2, 1912, 1.

39. Hospital and Health Board, "Contagious and Infectious Disease Reported," *Monthly Report of the Hospital and Health Board, Kansas City, Missouri* 6, no. 5 (May 1912); Hospital and Health Board, "Contagious Diseases Reported for the Year, 1912–1913," *Fifth Annual Report of the Hospital and Health Board of Kansas City, Missouri, for Fiscal Year April 16, 1912, to April 21, 1913* (Kansas City, MO: Hospital and Health Board, 1913), 87.

40. Hospital and Health Board, *Fourth Annual Report of the Hospital and Health Board of Kansas City, Missouri, for Fiscal Year April 17, 1911, to April 15, 1912, Inclusive* (Kansas City, MO: Hospital and Health Board, 1912), 106.

41. Ibid., 108.

42. Ibid., 23.

43. Dr. George R. Pipkin, "Report of Contagious Diseases," Hospital and Health Board, *Fourth Annual Report of the Hospital and Health Board of Kansas City, Missouri, for Fiscal Year April 17, 1911, to April 15, 1912, Inclusive* (Kansas City, MO: Hospital and Health Board, 1912), 148.

44. Arthur H. Parmelee, "Epidemic Cerebrospinal Meningitis," *Journal of the American Medical Association* 60, no. 9 (March 1, 1913): 659.

45. Ibid., 661.

46. "A Hospital, but No Furniture; Funds Are Lacking to Equip the City's New Isolation Building," *Kansas City Star*, July 27, 1912, 2.

A SERUM FARM FOR KANSAS CITY, AUGUST 1912–JULY 1913

O n Sunday, August 4, 1912, two and one-half weeks after Dr. Luscher had discharged his last cerebrospinal meningitis patient from the Kansas City General Hospital, Dr. Sophian, in New York City, boarded a train headed for Kansas City. Dr. Sophian's purpose in returning to Kansas City was to found with Dr. Frank Hall a Kansas City serum farm and laboratory to manufacture biologics for distribution in the midwestern and southwestern states.[1] The new biologics enterprise was hailed as "the greatest scientific project ever launched in Kansas City and the only one of its kind west of New York City's Rockefeller and Research Laboratories."[2] The new enterprise went by several names, including the Sophian-Hall-Alexander Laboratory, the Sophian-Hall-Alexander Laboratories, the Sophian-Hall-Alexander Biologic Company, and the Sophian-Hall-Alexander Biologic Laboratories.[3] Accompanying Dr. Sophian on the train were twenty-six-year-old Mr. Elliot Richie Alexander,[4] a chemist, and thirty-seven-year-old Thomas Deaken, a laboratory animal caretaker.[5] Both men were formerly employed by the Research Laboratory of the New York City Board of Health.

The Sophian-Hall-Alexander Laboratory procured the use of the Le Forest Farm at Eighty-Seventh Street and Wornall Road, south of the Kansas City limits,[6] and erected a barn for twelve horses.[7] Finding twelve healthy horses to purchase presented a challenge because a fatal horse epidemic of unknown etiology was rampant in the state of Kansas in August 1912.[8] As soon as he could acquire healthy horses, Dr. Sophian began immunizing them, because the production of high-quality sera required repetitive inoculations of killed and live cultures over many weeks and months, and the projected need for antimeningitis serum for the upcoming winter (1912–1913) was high. Recall that Dr. Hall had expressed deep concern to Dr. Sophian over inventorying an adequate supply of the serum for the upcoming winter, because the supply of the serum had failed during the height of the Kansas City cerebrospinal meningitis epidemic in late March and early April 1912.

The Sophian-Hall-Alexander Laboratory occupied an entire floor at 1208 Wyandotte Street in the heart of the business district of Kansas City.[6] The partners installed expensive equipment they had purchased on the East Coast of the United States and in Europe.[6, 9] Their initial investment in the enterprise was $30,000.[6] Dr. Hall continued to operate his American Biologic Company separately from the Sophian-Hall-Alexander Laboratory. Recall that Dr. Hall's laboratory was located in the nearby Gloyd Building.[9]

Dr. Sophian rented a flat in a three-story brick residential building at 2107 Linwood Boulevard, east of The Paseo and a block south of Thirty-First Street.[10] He next completed applications for federal licenses[11] to manufacture and sell across state lines the following biologics: diphtheria antitoxin; antigonococcic serum; antimeningococcic serum (antimeningitis serum); antistreptococcic serum; anti-rabic virus vaccine; bacterial vaccines, including Meningo-Bacterin (i.e., meningococcal vaccine); and normal serum.[12] The US Treasury required a separate federal license for each biologic and granted each license only after a federal agent visited a biologics' enterprise to confirm a company's compliance with regulations, such as maintaining sanitary premises that presented no menace to the people who worked or lived on or near the premises.

On Saturday, August 17, 1912, Dr. Sophian and Dr. Black published "Prophylactic Vaccination against Epidemic Meningitis" in the *Journal of the American Medical Association*. The article detailed their experiments in Dallas, Texas; promoted the efficacy and safety of the meningococcal vaccine across the nation; and urged physicians to use the vaccine to prevent cerebrospinal meningitis.[13]

In the same issue of the *Journal of the American Medical Association* (August 17, 1912), Dr. Hall published the following announcement: "Serum Farm and Laboratory for Kansas City— Dr. Frank J. Hall, Kansas City, has decided to establish a serum farm near the city and a laboratory in a downtown building, at which antitoxins and sera of various kinds will be manufactured. Drs. Abraham Sophian, Elliott [*sic*] R. Alexander and Mr. Thomas Deaken, all of New York City, are associated with Dr. Hall in his enterprise."[14]

On Monday, August 19, 1912, Dr. Luscher resigned as superintendent of the Kansas City General Hospital, where he had served for more than two grueling years.[15-17] He said he and the Hospital and Health Board members were parting as friends without ill feelings, the Kansas City General Hospital superintendent job was arduous, and he was glad of the opportunity for a rest. Under his leadership, the Kansas City General Hospital became recognized as one of the most efficient municipal institutions in the country.[15] The medical attending physicians and interns of the Kansas City General Hospital honored Dr. Luscher in a farewell dinner at the Hotel Savoy in Kansas City on Friday, August 30, 1912.[18] Dr. Luscher was fifty-four years old and would live ten more years.

On Tuesday, August 27, 1912, the Hospital and Health Board appointed Dr. Rush English Castelaw[19] to replace Dr. Luscher as superintendent of the Kansas City General Hospital.[20] Dr. Castelaw was trained as a pharmacist before earning his medical diploma from Kansas City Medical College. He also performed postgraduate work in neurology at the University of Pennsylvania and at the Neurological Hospital in New York City.[19] On Wednesday, August 28, 1912, the Hospital and Health Board appointed Dr. Sophian as a general consultant in medicine and contagious diseases at the Kansas City General Hospital.[21] His degree of involvement at the hospital is unknown.

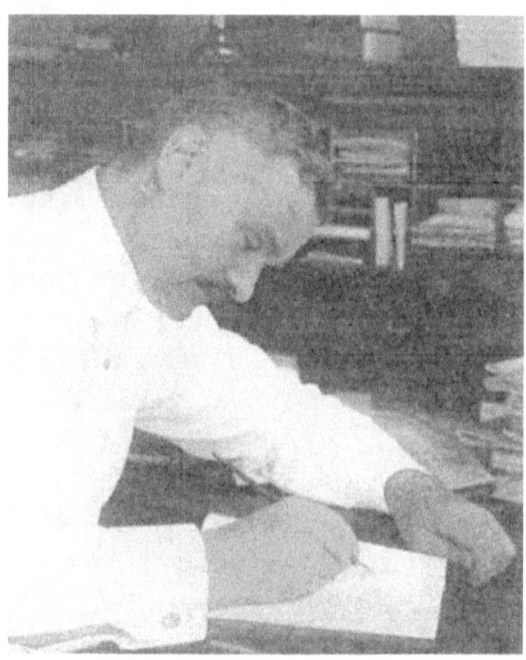

Dr. Rush E. Castelaw (1870–1970), 1912. The photographer is unknown. The image was scanned from the *Medical Herald* 31, no. 9 (September 1912), 472.

The numbers were low for new cases of, and deaths from, cerebrospinal meningitis in Kansas City in August, September, October, November, and December 1912: in those months, there were three cases and three deaths, one case and three deaths, two cases and one death, six cases and three deaths, and five cases and five deaths, respectively.[22] The weather during these five months was "wonderfully mild and pleasant and most favorable for all farm work and was never more so for feeding operations."[23] On December 31, 1912, a Missouri weather forecaster said, "Fair weather with moderate temperatures is all that's in sight ... A year ago, today there was three inches of snow on the ground [and] the mercury slid down to 3 degrees below zero."[24] The high and low temperatures on December 31, 1912, in Kansas City were forty-seven and thirty-five degrees Fahrenheit.[24]

On Saturday, December 7, 1912, Dr. Wheeler exuded optimism for the health of Kansas City: "I have never known Kansas City to be so free from sickness at this season before. There is no prevailing disease at all unless we might class the mild form of catarrhal influenza as one. There is some of that, but it is not at all widespread. I can truthfully say that we are entirely free from disease." Dr. Wheeler attributed the city's healthfulness to "the delightful autumn weather."[25]

During early December 1912, the Sophian-Hall-Alexander Laboratory announced its grand opening in a full-page advertisement in the *Medical Herald*:[26]

The Sophian-Hall-Alexander Laboratory wishes to announce to the medical profession that after several months of preparation it has its Biological preparations ready for distribution and use. Our Diphtheria Antitoxin and Anti-Meningitis Serum represent the last word in quality and containers.

The personnel of this Laboratory comprises [*sic*] the names of Dr. A. Sophian, already well known for his work on Epidemic Meningitis; Mr. E. R. Alexander, for several years his coworker as serum chemist in the New York Research Laboratory, in immediate charge of the Antitoxin department; and Dr. Frank J. Hall, who has been known here as a clinical pathologist for many years.

We wish the physicians of the Missouri Valley to feel a personal pride in furthering the interests of this distinctly ethical institution, to the end that we develop here a Laboratory for the production of serums and allied products that will rank with its model, the New York Research Laboratory.

Our full line of bacterins is most carefully prepared and sealed in ampoules without any addition of preservatives. Such a method of preparation insures the perfect specificity and potency of action. Special attention is directed to a faultless technique in the performance of the original Wassermann test [for syphilis]. The fee for this test has been reduced to ten dollars. A cordial invitation is extended [to] the profession to visit the Laboratory at 1208 Wyandotte Street. Kansas City, Mo.[26]

The company's products rapidly showed up in prescription drugstores in Kansas City.[27] In addition, the company published advertisements in other journals, such as the *Journal of the Oklahoma State Medical Association*.[28] Dr. Sophian also traveled to medical societies in Oklahoma and Kansas to lecture on cerebrospinal meningitis and notify medical society members of the availability of treatment for the disease.[29–32]

In December 1912, the *Medical Herald* published a paper on normal serum therapy written and read by Dr. Sophian in October 1912 before the Kansas City Academy of Medicine. In his paper, Dr. Sophian championed normal serum, "used from time immemorial," as one of the most valuable agents to treat surface wounds and suppurations, stomach and duodenal ulcerations, uterine inflammation, bladder infections, hemorrhage (in hemorrhagic diseases), nutritional disturbance, and sepsis. Human serum, said Dr. Sophian, was far preferable to alien sera, such as horse or rabbit sera, which could produce a serum sickness. However, human serum was difficult to obtain, whereas horse serum was readily available and in large quantities.[33]

After presenters read their papers before the Kansas City Academy of Medicine, audience members commented on the content of the papers. The *Medical Herald* published these comments and the presenters' responses to the same. Dr. Hall and Dr. Edwin Henry Schorer[34] made the following comments about Dr. Sophian's paper on normal serum therapy:

Dr. Hall: To me the whole proposition [efficacy of normal serum to reduce inflammation] is mysterious. The result of many of our experiments show valuable things that we cannot explain ... During the past few months, our laboratory furnished to a number of doctors, a large amount of rabbit's serum. Rabbit's serum has worked beautifully in hemorrhagic measles. This serum, it seems, whips up something in some sort of a way that gets results. I do not think there is any immunity established from horse serum. I think it is due the proteid products injected, metabolism is increased, and all processes are increased in their action, and as time goes on, we will find more of the value of alien serum and its stimulations ...

As far as serum sickness is concerned, I saw much of this during our last epidemic of meningitis, but when rashes developed, we did not stop. It is alarming, yet, I do not think it leaves permanent injury. What I did observe was, when serum was given in small doses, there was more serum sickness, than where it was given in large doses. I think it is a bad idea to give small doses of even diphtheria antitoxin. Here our experiments show good results from therapeutic measures we cannot explain, but why stand back because we cannot explain their action. Why wait till your patient is dead? I get tired of working on the dead myself. On many of the severe diseases, your chemical drugs help, but you do not have time to wait for their action. You want something that acts quick. Serum is the only thing you have at hand that does work quick. Of course, when we know the cause of our trouble, we can use the specific serum, but when you cannot diagnose the causative agent, use some serum that will bring about this stimulation and give results.[33]

Dr. Edwin Henry Schorer: Very frequently of course, we know in trying to immunize individuals, we have difficulty so far as curative action is concerned. Some of these difficulties come from the fact we are unable to get the antibody to the seat of infection, and for this reason we resort to various measures. We may resort to incision of an abscess. May apply the antibody to the area of infection, as in meningitis, or in tetanus, and then we also get the antibody to the part by some method of hyperemia, as rubefacients, etc. ... I realize there are certain diseases where normal horse serum is going to do good, but if we are going to use it without diagnosis, we are going backward. We should always make a diagnosis first, if at all possible. Then, perhaps if we cannot, then use the normal serum. We are taking a step backward to simply give a shot of this without first making a diagnosis. If we can get results with the normal serum, then we should get results surely with the antiserum.

In regard to serum disease. I do not know how many of you ever had this. I have had it. It is not a "cinch." It is possible to have sudden death of your patient from administering serum. I saw a man in Milwaukee die very suddenly, and I do not believe we should ever use horse serum in an individual unless there is an indication. It does produce sickness many times, and I feel this is an objectionable feature.[33]

Dr. Sophian responded to Drs. Hall and Schorer as follows:

First in reply to Dr. Schorer's remarks. It goes without saying that there must be a proper indication for any remedy, whether it be a drug or a serum, before it is used. Therefore of course, accurate diagnosis must first be made. I have seen a great many cases of serum sickness, but certainly do not consider it an objection to the use of serum in important cases ... In regard to anaphylaxis. True anaphylaxis is very rare. In important cases the uncommon danger of anaphylaxis shock must not be considered. In the epidemic of meningitis at Dallas a large number of cases had been sensitized with normal serum at some previous time. In no case did anaphylaxis occur, though serum sickness was quite frequent but apparently caused no serious damage. During the epidemic I advised the use of the sera as a temporary protection, especially in those who were intimately exposed to the disease. One of these immunized [people] developed meningitis about two months later. The intraspinal administration of serum caused no disturbance. In known cases of sensitization to foreign serum, it may be wise as a safeguard to administer a small dose subcutaneously at first before the larger doses are administered.[33]

On Wednesday, December 18, 1912, the Hospital and Health Board instructed Dr. Castelaw to purchase furnishings for fifty beds of the contagious-diseases hospital (its capacity was seventy beds). The board's goal was to open the contagious-diseases hospital on Wednesday, January 1, 1913, theoretically in time for the possible recurrence of a cerebrospinal meningitis and other epidemics.[35]

In January 1913, the *Medical Herald* published "Epidemic Cerebrospinal Meningitis," written by Dr. Albert Ware Nash, the Dallas City health officer, during the Texas cerebrospinal meningitis epidemic in 1912.[36] Dr. Nash had presented his paper earlier, on Tuesday, October 8, 1912, before the Medical Association of the

Southwest during its meeting in Hot Springs, Garland County, Arkansas.[36] In his paper, Dr. Nash shared his experience with 450 cerebrospinal meningitis patients in Dallas during the first six months of 1912. [Based on Dallas's population of 92,000 in 1910,[37] the prevalence of cerebrospinal meningitis during the first six months of 1912 calculated to a whopping *48.9 cerebrospinal meningitis cases per 10,000 Dallas residents.*]

For treatment of cerebrospinal meningitis, Dr. Nash advocated strict isolation of afflicted individuals in a single place, e.g., the Dallas City Hospital, and the quarantine of healthy carriers until their noses and throats could be cleared of meningococci with the use of antiseptic sprays. Concerning the use of a meningococcal vaccine, Dr. Nash said, "I am not prepared to say that I believe vaccination is a sure preventive, but I shall certainly give it a fair trial should another epidemic threaten, and I am sure that if the required number of doses [three] of the vaccine are taken, there will be quite a little immunity established." He acknowledged that he personally had taken only two doses of the vaccine and one dose of subcutaneous antimeningitis serum during the Dallas epidemic from January to June 1912.[36]

Dr. Nash also agreed that antimeningitis serum was the acknowledged treatment for patients afflicted with cerebrospinal meningitis. However, he was "convinced that lumbar puncture alone does quite a little good, by means of relieving the pressure, for certainly 'tis the pressure that causes quite a few of the symptoms." He estimated that he had performed two thousand lumbar puncture procedures and described his technique in detail.[36]

On Wednesday, January 15, 1913, Dr. Sophian lectured on cerebrospinal meningitis to the members of the Buchanan-Andrews County Medical Society in the assembly hall of the public library in St. Joseph, Buchanan County, Missouri (about fifty miles north of Kansas City).[29] The *Medical Herald* published in the February 1913 issue a lengthy and rich synopsis of Dr. Sophian's lecture to the Buchanan-Andrews County Medical Society.[29] On Tuesday, January 21, 1913, Dr. Sophian and Dr. Hall both spoke at a meeting of the Wichita, Sedgwick County Medical Society in

Wichita, Sedgwick County, Kansas (two hundred miles southwest of Kansas City).[30] Dr. Hall spoke on the histopathology of syphilis, regaling the audience with images of clinical syphilis in humans. Dr. Sophian presented his cerebrospinal meningitis lecture.

On Wednesday, January 24, 1913, the State Board of Health of Missouri held its meeting at the Jefferson Hotel in St. Louis, Missouri. The four members present were Drs. Gustav Bernhard Schulz[38] (president), Foster Wand Burke,[39] Louis Edward Bunte, and Frank Baker Hiller (secretary). Dr. Hiller introduced a proposition to distribute via county health agencies the sera, vaccines, and other biologics prepared by the Sophian-Hall-Alexander Biologic Company [sic] of Kansas City, Missouri. The four members approved entering into a yearlong contract with the company. Dr. Hiller signed the contract on behalf of the State Board of Health of Missouri, while Mr. Alexander accepted the contract on behalf of the Sophian-Hall-Alexander Biologic Company.[40]

An excerpt from the contract read,

The Sophian-Hall-Alexander Biologic Company, doing business in Kansas City, MO., agrees to furnish sera and vaccine under the following conditions to the State Board of Health: We will keep your office constantly supplied with a stock of fresh sera and vaccine; we will bear the shipping expense of sending all sera from our laboratories to your office. We will furnish you with a telegraphic code so that in case of urgent demand sera and vaccine may be ordered from us by wire, and we will also pay the costs of such telegrams ... Meningitis serum will be supplied in two containers, each holding 15 c.c. or 30 c.c. to one package, with needles, etc., all packed securely in a wooden box for shipment. The price per package to $1.50 for the sera and $1.00 for the containers and apparatus; a total of $2.50 for the complete package.[40]

During January 1913, there were ten cases of cerebrospinal meningitis and six deaths from the disease in Kansas City, according to the Hospital and Health Board.[22] The Kansas City weather in January 1913 was fair, mild, and dry. The highs and lows for Kansas City on January 14, 1913, were thirty-nine and twenty-three degrees, respectively, with predictions for a warming trend with rain.[41] During the last week of January 1913, the high and low temperatures were in the fifties and forties, respectively. By contrast, the high and low temperatures on January 30, 1912, during the cerebrospinal meningitis epidemic of 1912, had hovered in the thirties and teens (Fahrenheit).[41]

On Friday, February 7, 1913, Dr. Wade Hampton Frost, the United States Public Health physician who previously had published a primer[42] on meningococcal meningitis (January 1912) in the *Public Health Reports*, as noted above, issued a somewhat harsh and unsolicited critique[43] of Drs. Sophian and Black's paper "Prophylactic Vaccination against Epidemic Meningitis," which they had published six months earlier, on August 17, 1912.[13] In his critique, Dr. Frost alleged that Dr. Sophian and Dr. Black had failed to demonstrate convincingly the efficacy of the meningococcal vaccine. He also listed the untenable (in his opinion) risks and costs of wholesale meningococcal vaccination and strongly advised against the wholesale use of meningococcal vaccination except "in communities where the disease was epidemic, or where an epidemic seemed likely to occur, especially of physicians and nurses caring for patients with the disease."[43] In his earlier primer, Dr. Frost had written, "The high mortality of cerebrospinal meningitis, its peculiarly distressing clinical course, and the frequency of most serious after-effects render it imperative that *every possible measure be taken to protect the public from its ravages*" [emphasis added].[42]

During February 1913, there were ten new cases of cerebrospinal meningitis and twelve deaths from the disease, according to the Hospital and Health Board.[22] The weather continued remarkably mild. One observer wrote,

The 1913 winter has been a beautiful fall or early spring, except for three days early in January. Only five inches of snow have fallen during the entire season. The days have been warm enough for the men to go about without their overcoats and the women have discarded their furs ... Kansas was expecting an unusually hard winter and was prepared for it. But there were only three days of extreme cold. But even those three days brought a temperature record never before reaching in some parts of the state.[44]

On Monday, March 3, 1913, Dr. Arthur H. Parmelee published "Epidemic Cerebrospinal Meningitis" in the *Journal of the American Medical Association* less than a year after he battled the disease as an intern at the Kansas City General Hospital. In his review, Dr. Parmelee noted the occasional occurrence of respiratory failure in several patients. Physicians seldom could revive these patients, although their patients' hearts continued to beat strongly and rhythmically for some time. In one case, staff performed artificial respiration for fifty minutes, as the heart beat strongly until within a few minutes of the end. Five patients recovered from the respiratory paralysis with the aid of artificial respiration. Physicians noted cardiac paralysis alone in two cases. Dr. Parmelee did not posit a cause for the occasional cardiorespiratory failure witnessed in patients with cerebrospinal meningitis.[45]

On Sunday, March 17, 1913, Dr. Simon Pendleton Kramer[46] of Cincinnati, Hamilton County, Ohio, reported to his colleagues of the Cincinnati Academy of Medicine his belief that antimeningitis serum was responsible for the recent deaths of five children at the Cincinnati City Hospital. Each of the five children had died within five minutes of an intraspinal injection of the serum. Two other children had survived but only with strenuous resuscitation efforts. Dr. Kramer attributed the deaths to the presence of tricresol, a germicide commonly used as a serum preservative.[47] Dr. Kramer claimed that tricresol was harmless in adults but fatal in children, reasoning that the central canal of the spinal cord in children was still patent, thus permitting the tricresol to find its way quickly to the medulla oblongata of the brain to cause almost instantaneous death.[48] He referenced Dr. Parmelee's findings about respiratory deaths in a number of patients, as noted above.[49] Dr. Kramer's allegation about tricresol reverberated in newspapers around the United States.[50]

Dr. Flexner roundly defended the safety of the tricresol in his antimeningitis serum recipe; mentioned that Dr. Sophian, the physician who probably had had the largest single experience in administering antimeningitis serum (1,500 injections), never had had a single incident like that described by Dr. Kramer; and suggested slow injection of the antimeningitis serum to avoid suddenly increasing intracranial pressure, which could cause respiratory failure.[51] Investigators at the Research Laboratory of the New York City Board of Health, the source of the antimeningitis serum used by Dr. Kramer, studied the tricresol toxicity issue and replaced tricresol with chloroform as the serum preservative beginning in 1914.[52]

During March 1913, there were seventeen cases of cerebrospinal meningitis and sixteen deaths from the disease in Kansas City.[22] The weather in March 1913 was mild, with one major widespread storm midmonth that produced heavy rain or snow in Missouri.[53]

On March 12, 1913, the new contagious-diseases hospital finally opened.[54] However, Dr. Castelaw admitted smallpox patients to the isolation ward of the Old Hospital instead of to the new contagious-diseases hospital. A well-to-do female patient with a light case of smallpox complained about her placement in the Old Hospital. Dr. Castelaw responded, "Conditions as this patient described them do not exist at the old city hospital. She is nervous and cranky and we expected her to complain of her surroundings. The floors there are clean and she gets good treatment. The other patients in the room are as nice girls as you would care to meet." He added, "The contagious-diseases hospital has wards for measles, diphtheria, scarlet fever, and meningitis. I do not know why smallpox was omitted, but it was and we'll have to put up with it." Other physicians at the Kansas City General Hospital countered Dr. Castelaw, saying they were caring for the meningitis and scarlet fever patients in the Kansas City General Hospital, not in the contagious-diseases hospital.[54]

On Saturday, March 22, 1913, Dr. Castelaw said that people "could be frightened into an epidemic" and told them, "The main thing is to keep a level head. A great deal of damage can be done by saying there is an epidemic when there is none. There is absolutely nothing to this meningitis scare. Right here in Kansas City we have a disease that is more fatal, yet persons pay no attention to it. Physicians have reported 65 cases of pneumonia, out of which there have been 50 deaths. Yet I do not consider that an epidemic in a city of this size." He continued, "We have one case of cerebrospinal meningitis at the hospital now and never have we had more than five cases at one time during the winter. It is strictly a winter disease."[55] However, on Thursday, April 3, 1913, Dr. Castelaw acknowledged the presence of six patients with cerebrospinal meningitis in the Kansas City General Hospital.[56]

During April 1913, there were eleven new cases of cerebrospinal meningitis and fifteen deaths from the disease in Kansas City.[22] The weather in April 1913 was so mild generally that Judge J. L. McCurdy, a Missouri farmer, planted his corn on Saturday, April 19, 1913.[57]

On Wednesday, April 2, 1913, and again on Monday, April 28, 1913, Dr. Sophian lectured on cerebrospinal meningitis to medical groups in Emporia, Kansas, and Muskogee, Oklahoma, respectively.[31-32] Muskogee physicians remembered him as "the physician who, more than anyone else, helped check the big meningitis epidemic in Texas [in 1912] by showing the Texas physicians the uses of serum in the treatment of meningitis." They also recalled that the death rate from the disease fell from 80 percent to less than 50 percent after the introduction of the serum treatment and the training of the physicians by Dr. Sophian in its use. Dr. Sophian said in his lecture, "Meningitis is a disease but slightly more dangerous than typhoid, when treated with the serum. The results that have been obtained by the use of the serum treatment prove the immense benefit it has been in the treatment of meningitis."[31]

Also, in April 1913, Dr. Sophian published his book titled *Epidemic Cerebrospinal Meningitis*.[58] The *Medical Herald* noted, "Dr. A. Sophian has written the only book devoted to epidemic cerebrospinal meningitis. It is just now off the press by the Mosby Publishing Company, St. Louis. The *Herald* has been asked to review the work and will do soon."[59]

In the April 1913 issue of the *Journal of the Missouri State Medical Association*, the editors acclaimed the Sophian-Hall-Alexander Biologic Company, noting,

> Missouri, the public at large, and the profession of the midwest and southwest are fortunate indeed, over the recent establishment in Kansas City of a modern and thoroughly equipped laboratory for the scientific investigation of pathologic and therapeutic problems, and the manufacture of biologic products. Kansas City on account of its location in western Missouri, and as the gateway to a populous southwest territory with vast agricultural and animal resources, occupies a position, medically, of vast importance, making imminent and absolutely essential the establishment here of such a laboratory for purposes of research and experimentation along lines of preventive and curative medicine.[60]

The article continued,

> The men represented and in control of this laboratory are known to the American profession as scientific and practical. Dr. A. Sophian comes from the New York Research Laboratory ... Mr. E. R. Alexander is an expert chemist and was an associate with Dr. Sophian in his work in the New York Research Laboratory ... Dr. Frank J. Hall, as a pathologist

and bacteriologist, and as a practical laboratory man, needs no introduction to the profession ... A visit to the laboratory in Kansas City and to the farm at Waldo [a small settlement on the southern fringes of Kansas City][61] will convince one of the complete and extensive equipment, and of products most perfectly prepared and carefully preserved. It is very evident that neither time nor expense is being spared in the improvement and perfection of their various biologic products ... Such men and such institutions are a necessity to all large centers of population and should prove an asset. It is to be hoped that this modern biologic laboratory so conveniently located may be recognized, visited and received the support it so well merits from the profession of Missouri and surrounding territory.[60]

On April 15, 1913, the Council on Pharmacy and Chemistry of the American Medical Association[62] approved the following biologics produced by the Sophian-Hall-Alexander Biologic Laboratories as new and nonofficial remedies: acne vaccine, antimeningococcus serum [antimeningitis serum], bacillus coli vaccine, serum antidiphthericum and antidiphtheric globulines, gonococcus vaccine, meningococcus vaccine, pneumococcus vaccine, bacillus pyocyaneus vaccine, staphylococcus vaccines (polyvalent staphylococcus vaccine and polyvalent staphylo-acne vaccine), streptococcus vaccine, and typhoid vaccine.

In addition, the Council on Pharmacy and Chemistry of the American Medical Association notified readers about the following transfer of agency: the Sophian-Hall-Alexander Laboratories now manufactured the antirabic vaccine formerly manufactured by the American Biologic Company (Dr. Hall's laboratory).[63] The Council on Pharmacy and Chemistry based its acceptance of these products largely on evidence supplied by the manufacturer or his agent and in part on investigation made by or under the direction of the council. The council counseled readers that the acceptance of a product did not necessarily mean a recommendation, but so far as known, the product complied with the rules adopted by the council.[62]

In late April 1913, the Hospital and Health Board members began the compilation of the *Fifth Annual Report of the Hospital and Health Board of Kansas City for Fiscal Year April 16, 1912, to April 21, 1913, Inclusive.* In it, Dr. Castelaw and Dr. Wheeler presented their data on the second year of the cerebrospinal meningitis epidemic, 1912–1913.

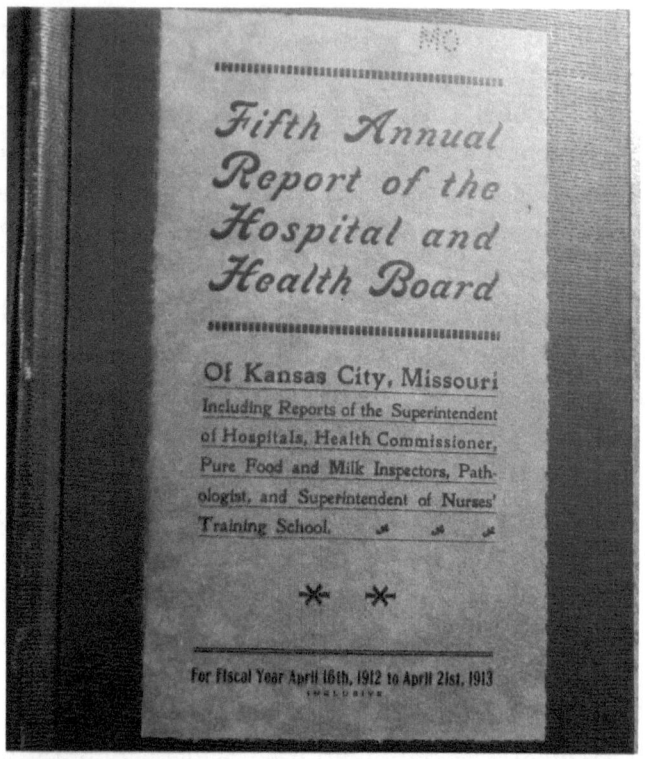

Front cover of the *Fifth Annual Report of the Hospital and Health Board of Kansas City, Missouri, for Fiscal Year April 15th, 1912 to April 21st, 1913.* Photographer: M. O'Leary.

In the *Fifth Annual Report of the Hospital and Health Board,* Dr. Castelaw reported 119 cases of cerebrospinal meningitis admitted to the Kansas City General Hospital and 14 cases to the Old Hospital, totaling 133 cerebrospinal meningitis patients admitted to the city's two public hospitals during the second year of the epidemic (1912–1913). Dr. Castelaw said that the death data for the Kansas City General Hospital and the Old Hospital were 40 percent (forty-eight deaths) and 29 percent (four deaths), respectively. Dr. Castelaw added, "It will be noted that the death rate is lower than that of the first year of the epidemic [1911–1912] for the cases treated at the hospital, viz.: 52 percent. This is due to the fact that cases were sent to us earlier and that no difficulty was experienced in obtaining and administering serum. Also, that the virulence of the disease has a tendency to weaken year to year [sic]."[64]

In the *Fifth Annual Report of the Hospital and Health Board*, Dr. Wheeler reported 121 cases of cerebrospinal meningitis in Kansas City during the second year of the epidemic (1912–1913), with a death rate of 94 percent (114 deaths). He was stunned by the data, writing, "The death rate, as you see, was appalling, and I have no way of knowing just why it should be so high other than the fact that the disease attacked those that had been greatly reduced physically and long carriers of the germ. Early last fall [1912], I districted the rooming house section of our city and required a thorough cleaning of all rooming houses, boarding houses, small hotels, and many homes in the northern section of the city."[65]

In summary, the number of cases of cerebrospinal meningitis counted during the second year of the epidemic was less than one-quarter (around 120 cases) of the number of cases (414 cases) counted by the Hospital and Health Board during the first year of the epidemic (1911–1912). The prevalence of cerebrospinal meningitis dropped from around *16.6 cerebrospinal meningitis cases per 10,000 Kansas City residents* between January 1, 1912, and June 1, 1912, to around *4.8 cerebrospinal meningitis cases per 10,000 Kansas City residents* between May 1, 1912, and April 30, 1913.

In May 1913, new cases of the disease continued to appear sporadically in Kansas City, much to the dismay of the health department officials and private physicians: i.e., seven cases of cerebrospinal meningitis and five deaths from the disease. In June 1913, there were four cases of cerebrospinal meningitis and four deaths from the disease.[66] The weather in May 1913 was rainy and warm generally, with highs in the fifties and sixties.[67] Weather in June 1913 warmed further, portending an unusually hot summer.[68]

In June 1913, Dr. Sophian's *Epidemic Cerebrospinal Meningitis* drew complimentary reviews in a number of medical and public health journals.[69] For example, the *Medical Herald* book reviewer wrote,

> This is one of the few books actually needed to be added to the present day medical literature. It's the one American volume devoted to Epidemic Meningitis. Its contents are fresh from scientific studies of the research laboratory and the practical field work of our recent epidemic. The central west owes much to the author for his devotion and personal sacrifice in the epidemic zone work in the time of need and the profession is now favored by the condensed results of his labor. The six chapters are: Etiology, Symptomatology, Laboratory Diagnosis, Complications, Studies on Blood-Pressure in Meningitis, and Treatment.[70]

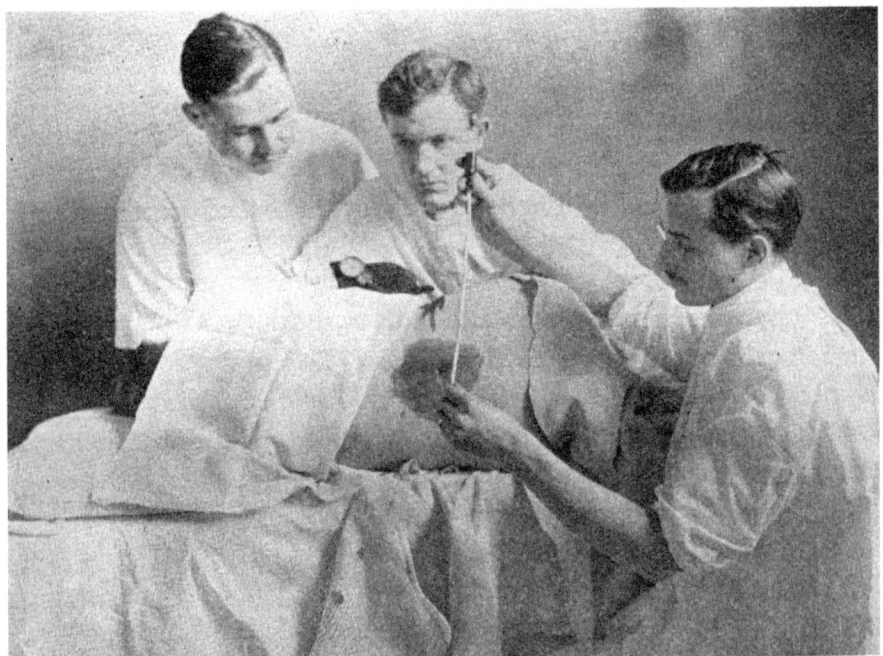

Image of Dr. Abraham Sophian (1885–1957) (seated on the far right) while performing a lumbar puncture procedure and infusing Flexner antimeningitis serum by gravity, circa 1912–1913. The original caption to the image says, "Fig. XIV. This picture illustrates the operation of lumbar puncture and the technique in injecting the antimeningitis serum. The patient is lying on his left side over the right flexing the hips on his abdomen and bending his head forward. The skin at the site of the operation has been painted with tincture of iodine. The site of the operation is draped off with sterile towels. The needle has been inserted at the level of the crest of the ileum, which is marked with tincture of iodine. The assistant at the head of the patient is taking blood pressure observations. The serum is being injected by gravity." The photographer is unknown. The image was scanned from Abraham Sophian, *Epidemic Cerebrospinal Meningitis* (St. Louis, MO: C. V. Mosby, 1913), 171.

The book reviewer for the *American Journal of Public Health* wrote,

> It is a pleasure to review a book on cerebrospinal meningitis by one who has done so large an amount of original investigation in this field, as Doctor Sophian. Unlike many present-day writers, this monograph is not a mere collection of statements collected from the writings of others. What data have been collected from the literature are invariably combined with a well-reasoned analysis which leaves the reader in no doubt as to the author's belief or disbelief in their correctness ... Owing to the excellence of the entire work, it is difficult to pick out any one particular part of the monograph for special commendation.[71]

In July 1913, the *Public Health Reports* reported that the Sophian-Hall-Alexander Laboratory was an establishment now licensed by the US Treasury Department to propagate and sell the following biologics: diphtheria antitoxin, antigonococcic serum, antimeningococcic serum (antimeningitis serum), antistreptococcic serum, antirabic virus [*sic*], normal horse serum, and bacterial vaccines.[72] In less than one year, Dr. Sophian, Dr. Hall, Mr. Alexander, and Mr. Deaken had established a first-class biologics company on the western frontier of the United States.

On Tuesday, July 1, 1913, Dr. Castelaw closed the contagious-diseases hospital because of a lack of patients with contagious diseases who required hospitalization. Kansas City had only one person with smallpox at the time, whom Dr. Castelaw placed at the Old Hospital. Between Wednesday, March 12, 1913, and the closing of the hospital on Tuesday, July 1, 1913, patients with the following contagious diseases received their care in the contagious-diseases hospital: cerebrospinal meningitis (19 patients), diphtheria (22), scarlet fever (6), measles (136), whooping cough (4), and scabies (5). The largest number of patients cared for at any one time in the contagious-diseases hospital was forty-nine. On Thursday, July 10, 1913, Dr. Castelaw remarked that the health situation in Kansas City was "just as good or better than any other summer."[73]

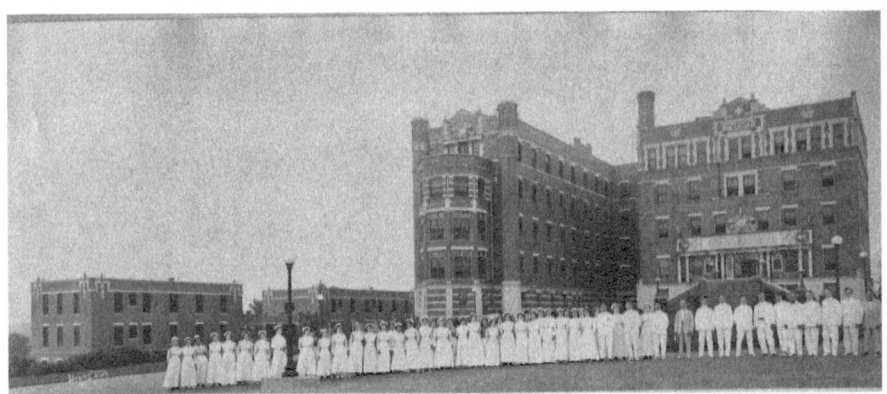

Contagious-diseases hospital (left side of image) of the Kansas City General Hospital (right side of image), 1914. The image was photographed looking toward the east, with the contagious-diseases building to the north. The hospital staff stand in front of the hospital. The image is courtesy of the Truman Medical Center Archives, Kansas City, Mo.

During July 1913, there was one new case of cerebrospinal meningitis and one death from the disease in Kansas City.[67] The weather in July 1913 in Kansas City was hot and dry.[74]

CHAPTER 6 NOTES

1. "Anti-Toxin Farm at Kansas City: Scientists Will Supply World with Serum; Dr. Sophian of New York, Who Helped Stamp Out Meningitis There, One of the Members," *Chillicothe Morning Constitution*, August 5, 1912, 1.

2. "Anti-Toxin Farm at Kansas City: Scientists Will Supply World with Serum; Dr. Sophian of New York, Who Helped Stamp Out Meningitis There, One of the Members," *Chillicothe Morning Constitution*, August 5, 1912, 1.

3. "Medical News," *Medical Herald* 32, no. 11 (November 1913): 431.

4. Mr. Elliot Ritchie Alexander (1886–1939) was born in Brooklyn, New York, as the eldest of the four children of James Ritchie Alexander (1858–1915), a hat maker, and Sarah Amanda Vanderhoef (1859–1922). Elliot earned his bachelor's degree in chemistry from Columbia University in 1910, worked as a chemist at the Research Laboratory of the New York City Board of Health (1910–1912), and partnered with Dr. Abraham Sophian and Dr. Frank Hall to establish a serum farm and laboratory in Kansas City (1912–1914). He subsequently moved to New Brunswick, Middlesex County, New Jersey, to work as the research chemist for E. R. Squibbs Biological and Research Laboratories (1914–1918). He next returned with Dr. Sophian to Kansas City in 1918 and later moved to Orlando, Florida, to found the Tropical Vitamin Company and the Vitamin Company of America. The best-known product of his companies was the Vitabar, a candy fruit health product that contained "all the vitamins known to the world," including the citrus vitamins. He married Lena Weissenborn (1893–1953) sometime before 1917; they had two children. He died at the age of fifty-three years. See Wade W. Oliver, *The Man Who Lived for Tomorrow* (New York: E. P. Dutton, 1941), 304; William Hallock Park, "The New Activities of the Research Laboratory of the Department of Health of the City of New York," *Monthly Bulletin of the Department of Health* 1–2 (1911–1912): 57; "Elliot R. Alexander; Complete List of 600 Automobile Licenses Issued for 1914," *Central New Jersey Home News* (New Brunswick, NJ), February 21, 1914, 15; "Elliot R. Alexander; Many Drivers Licenses Have Been Issued by Walter Williamson," *Central New Jersey Home News*, February 28, 1914, 13; "Highland Park and Livingston Manor Notes," *Central New Jersey Home News*, June 2, 1914, 7; "Fined for Speeding," *Central New Jersey Home News*,

June 8, 1914, 1; and "Vitamin Bar Firm Showing Fine Growth; 25,000 Bars of Chocolate Covered Fruit Product Now Being Turned Out Daily," *Orlando Evening Star* (Orlando, Florida), November 16, 1930, 2.

5. Thomas Joseph Deaken (1875–1947) was born in the Red Hook neighborhood of Brooklyn, New York, as the youngest of the four children of Thomas M. Deaken (1835–1878), a seaman, and Catherine Comber (1845–1923). Young Thomas's father was born in Whitehaven, England, and died in a hurricane southeast of Cape Hatteras, North Carolina, on December 10, 1878. His mother was born in Ireland. They married in 1864. Thomas J. Deaken worked as a janitor before joining the Research Laboratory as a laboratory assistant and animal caretaker around 1905. He married Margaret M. McHugh (1882–1963) in 1903; they had seven children between 1905 and 1921. Margaret might have accompanied Thomas to Kansas City in 1912, as one of their children (Marion) was born in Missouri in 1914. Their other six children were born in New York.

6. "To Battle Meningitis: Farm Is to Prevent Shortage in Necessary Serum," *Fort Wayne Sentinel* (Fort Wayne, IN), August 24, 1912, 13.

7. "Serum Farm a Menace? A Property Owner Protests against German Inoculation in the City," *Kansas City Star*, July 14, 1913, 4.

8. Kansas State Governor Walter Roscoe Stubbs (1858–1929) and Joseph Hooker Mercer (born in 1864), the state livestock sanitary commissioner, recruited Dr. Sophian to help them learn the elusive cause of the Kansas horse epidemic. As many as forty thousand of Kansas's one million horses (roughly equaling the number of humans in the state) died after developing a listless, dull, and expressionless appearance; standing in one position; staggering when forced to walk; and showing difficulty drinking water due to paralysis of the muscles used in swallowing. Dr. Sophian eventually diagnosed a virus as the cause of the disease, but Kansas horse experts rejected his assessment. His diagnosis subsequently was proven correct. See Richard F. Raugewitz, "The Horse Disease in Kansas, 1912–1913," *Emporia State Research Studies* 20, no, 2 (December 1917): 1–20; "Horse Plague Disastrous; Over 40 Died in Barton County Last Thursday Night; Stubbs Wires Taft; Disease Appeared in Ness County Three Weeks Ago; Nature of Disease Not Yet Determined; Burning Dead Animals," *Weekly Gazette Globe*, August 31, 1912, 1; and R. A. McIntosh, "Equine Encephalomyelitis from a Clinician's

Point of View," *Canadian Journal of Comparative Medicine* 2, no. 8 (August 1938): 223.

9. "A Serum Farm in Kansas City," *Medical Herald* 31, no. 9 (September 1912): 471.

10. *US City Directories*, 1912, Kansas City for Abraham Sophian, 32B. The building is still standing as of this writing.

11. "Biological Products: Establishments Licensed for the Propagation and Sale of Viruses, Serums, Toxins, and Analogous Products," *Public Health Reports* 28, no. 28 (July 11, 1913): 1447.

12. Dr. Sophian postulated that all artificial hyperemias, such as heat baths or heat packs, acted by bringing normal serum in excess to the stimulated area. See Abraham Sophian, "Normal Serum Therapy," *Medical Herald* 31, no. 12 (December 1912): 615–20.

13. Abraham Sophian and James Harvey Black, "Prophylactic Vaccination against Epidemic Meningitis," *Journal of the American Medical Association* 59, no. 7 (August 17, 1912): 527–32.

14. "Medical News: Missouri: Serum Farm and Laboratory for Kansas City," *Journal of the American Medical Association* 59, no. 7 (August 17, 1912): 553.

15. "City Hospital Head Quits; 'I Was Asked to Resign,' Dr. L. W. Luscher Says; The Resignation of the General Hospital Superintendent Is Regarded as Another Turn in the Political Head—'No Hard Feelings,' Luscher Says," *Kansas City Star*, August 18, 1912, 2.

16. "New Head for Hospital; Dr. R. E. Castelaw Slated to Succeed Doctor Luscher; City Hall Gossip Attributes the Ousting of the Present Incumbent to a Tiff with W. P. Motley—Negro Internes the Contention," *Kansas City Star*, August 19, 1912, 3.

17. The alleged reason for Dr. Luscher's resignation was his alleged insistence on the dismissal of African American interns for lack of merit at the Kansas City General Hospital No. 2 (the Old Hospital). The newly renovated Old Hospital had been turned over to the African American citizens of Kansas City in 1911. In 1912, a petition signed by fourteen of the eighteen members of the visiting staff of the Old Hospital recommended that the Hospital and Health Board displace the African American interns at the Old Hospital by white interns because the former had failed to pass the competitive entrance examination. The test papers, which had been graded by six members of the staff who had prepared the questions, ranged from 30 to 65 percent out of a possible 100 percent. Seventy-five percent was the minimum acceptable mark. William Perry Motley,

the president of the Hospital and Health Board, obtained the test papers and submitted them to a second set of graders, declaring, "Just give me those papers. I will bring them back next week. I would like to know how a man can go to medical school four years, be graduated there and then make such grades." Physicians blinded to the identities of the test takers regraded the test papers, and four of the five African American interns received passing grades. "Hospital Retains Negro Internes; President of Health Board 'Puts One Over' on Surgeon Staff—Has Papers Regraded—Outside Doctors Rank Negro Applicants as Winners at Old Institution," *Washington Bee* (Washington, DC), August 24, 1912, 4; and "Afro-American Cullings," *Savannah Tribune* (Savannah, Georgia), September 21, 1912, 2.

18. "Farewell Dinner to Luscher; The Former Hospital Head Will Be the Guest of the Internes and Physicians," *Kansas City Star*, August 30, 1912, 5.

19. Dr. Rush English Castelaw (1870–1970) was born in Carrollton, Greene County, Illinois, as one of the six children of David Marion Castelaw (1836–1924), a blacksmith, and Josephine English (1837–1917). Rush Castelaw graduated from public high school in 1887; moved to Kansas City in 1888; earned his pharmacy degree from the Kansas City College of Pharmacy (established in 1885) in 1893; and opened a drugstore in the city. In 1902, he earned his medical diploma from the Kansas City Medical College, and he worked as a police surgeon in the Emergency Hospital in the basement of Kansas City City [*sic*] Hall from 1902 to 1907. He next took advanced work at the University of Pennsylvania (1909–1910). In 1910, he applied for the job of superintendent of the Kansas City General Hospital but lost out to Dr. Luscher. In 1911, he studied at the Neurological Hospital in New York City under Dr. Joseph Collins (1866–1950). He again applied for, and this time won, the job of superintendent of the Kansas City General Hospital (1912–1914). He subsequently became the superintendent of Wesley Hospital in Kansas City (during the later 1910s), the Christian Church Hospital of Kansas City (during the early 1920s), and the Decatur and Macon County Hospital in Illinois (during the late 1920s) before retiring. He served as secretary of the Jackson County Medical Society for two terms. In 1922, at the age of fifty-two years, he married Octavia H. Bierer (1891–1982); they had no children. He lived to be one hundred years old. See "Our Vice Presidents," *Journal of the Missouri State*

Medical Association 9 (July 1914–December 1914): 461; "News of the Month, Kansas City," *Medical Herald* 30, no. 6 (June 1911): 292; "A Hospital Head Tuesday," *Kansas City Star*, July 17, 1910, 4; and "Longevity Formula Takes Him to Age 95," *Sedalia Democrat*, April 12, 1964, 4.

20. "Kansas City General Hospital," *Medical Herald* 31, no. 9 (September 1912): 472; "New Head for Hospital; Dr. R. E. Castelaw Slated to Succeed Doctor Luscher; City Hall Gossip Attributes the Ousting of the Present Incumbent to a Tiff with W. P. Motley—Negro Internes the Contention," *Kansas City Star*, August 19, 1912, 3; and "New Hospital Head Today," *Kansas City Star*, August 27, 1912, 1.

21. "The General Hospital Staff; Physicians and Surgeons Named for the Year Beginning September 1," *Kansas City Star*, August 28, 1912, 3.

22. Hospital and Health Board, "Contagious and Infectious Diseases Reported," *Monthly Report of the Hospital and Health Board, Kansas City, Missouri* 7, no. 1 (January 1913); Hospital and Health Board, "Contagious and Infectious Diseases for the Year 1912–1913," *Fifth Annual Report of the Hospital and Health Board of Kansas City, Missouri, for Fiscal Year April 16, 1912, to April 21, 1913 Inclusive* (Kansas City, MO: Hospital and Health Board, 1913), 88.

23. "Big Kansas Wheat Area," *Kansas City Star*, December 31, 1912, 3.

24. "The Weather—Fair," *Kansas City Star*, December 31, 1912, 1.

25. "Feeling Fine, Thank You! Less Sickness at This Season Than in Years, Doctor Wheeler Says; Healthful Conditions Are Attributed to the Delightful Weather That Has Been Free from Violent Storm or Sudden Changes," *Kansas City Star*, December 7, 1912, 2.

26. "Announcement: The Sophian-Hall-Alexander Laboratory," *Medical Herald* 31, no. 12 (December 1912): 673.

27. For example, see "Hunter Brothers" advertisement, *Kansas City Star*, repeated on December 6, 13, 20, 1912, and January 3, 1913.

28. See "The Sophian-Hall-Alexander Laboratories," *Journal of the Oklahoma State Medical Association* 5, no. 3 (January 1913): 391. See also "Advertisements: Why Fear Rabies?" *Journal of the Missouri State Medical Association* 9, no. 12 (June 1913): vii.

29. "Epidemic Meningitis," *Medical Herald* 32, no. 2 (February 1913): 75–77, 86.

30. "Society Scintillations: Wichita, Sedgwick County Medical Society," *Medical Herald* 32, no. 2 (February 1913): 85.

31. "Medics: Listen to a Lecture by Dr. Sophian, the Man Who Conquored [*sic*] Meningitis in Dallas Last Year," *Muskogee Times-Democrat* (Muskogee, OK), April 28, 1913, 1.

32. "The Doctors' Meeting," *Emporia Gazette* (Emporia, KS), April 2, 1913, 4.

33. Abraham Sophian, "Normal Serum Therapy," *Medical Herald* 31, no. 12 (December 1912): 615–20.

34. Dr. Edwin "Teddy" Henry Schorer (1879–1966) was born in Plymouth, Sheboygan County, Wisconsin, as the eldest of the five children of Robert Rudolph Schorer (1849–1926), a merchandise proprietor and furniture store owner, and Bertha Wallschlaeger (1855–1935). Teddy Schorer earned his bachelor's degree from the University of Wisconsin (1902); spent one summer at the Rockefeller Institute for Medical Research under the aegis of Dr. Simon Flexner (1903); served as the pathologist and bacteriologist to the Thomas Wilson Sanitarium for Children in Baltimore (1904–1905); earned his medical degree from Johns Hopkins School of Medicine (1906); and earned his doctorate of public health from Harvard University (1912). He next worked for one year as a professor of parasitology and hygiene at the University of Missouri in Columbia, Boone County, Missouri. In 1913, he moved to Kansas City, where he practiced pediatrics for the next fifty years. He served two years in the US Army Laboratory at Fort Riley, where he was involved in the development and testing of an army meningococcal vaccine. He also served as the health director of Kansas City (1935–1940). He married Margaret M. Shrive (1886–1966) in 1910; they had one child. He married Annette Otto (1898–1989) in 1920. He died at the age of eighty-six years. He wrote and published *Vaccine and Serum Therapy* (St. Louis, MO: C. V. Mosby Company, 1913). *Harvard University Directory* (Cambridge, MA: Harvard University Press, 1913), 713; *General Catalogue of the Officers and Graduates of the University of Wisconsin 1849–1907* (Madison, WI: University of Wisconsin, 1907), 1902; and "Dr. E. H. Schorer Is Dead at 86," *Kansas City Times*, February 26, 1966, 1, 2.

35. "Contagion Hospital Ready January 1," *Kansas City Star*, December 18, 1912, 2.

36. Albert W. Nash, "'Epidemic Cerebrospinal Meningitis,' Official Transactions, Medical Association of the Southwest, Seventh Annual Session at Hot Springs, Ark., October 8–10, 1912," in *Medical Herald* 32, no. 1 (January 1913): 8–11.

37. *Texas Almanac: City Population History of Selected Cities, 1850–2000*, accessed December 8, 2017, https://texasalmanac.com/sites/default/files/images/CityPopHist%20web.pdf.

38. Dr. Gustav Bernhard Schulz (1870–1954) was born in Wittenberg, Perry County, Missouri, as one of the seven children of Dr. Frederick Bernhard Schulz (1828–1908) and Alwiena August Zedler (1838–1898). As a small child, he moved with his family across the Missouri River to Grande Tower, Jackson County, Illinois, to escape a smallpox epidemic. In 1876, his family moved to Cape Girardeau, Cape Girardeau County, Missouri. He attended St. Vincent College and the Normal School in Cape Girardeau before moving to St. Louis to work in a pharmacy. Next, he entered the Beaumont Hospital Medical College in St. Louis, where he earned his medical degree in 1892 at the age of twenty-two years. He served as an intern at the City Hospital of St. Louis; moved to Altenburg, Perry County, Missouri, to practice medicine for ten years; and took over his father's practice in Cape Girardeau in 1903. Governor Herbert S. Hadley, a close personal friend, appointed him to a four-year term on the State Board of Health of Missouri (1910–1914). Dr. Schulz studied at the Mayo Clinic in Rochester, Minnesota, where he befriended Drs. Charles and William Mayo. During their boat trips down the Mississippi River, they visited him in Cape Girardeau. Dr. Schulz married Alice Knight, a nurse, in 1916; they had no children. They converted their home in Cape Girardeau into a hospital. He died of heart disease at the age of eighty-three years. See Warren Schmidt, "Surgeon from Wittenberg," Lutheran Heritage Center and Museum, Perry County Lutheran Historical Society Missouri, accessed April 23, 2018, https://lutheranmuseum.com/2016/11/02/surgeon-from-wittenberg/.

39. Dr. Foster Wand Burke Sr. (1874–1935) possibly was born in Laclede, Linn County, Missouri, as one of the four children of Dr. John Lewis Burke (1847–1918) and Mary Frances Moss (1852–1932). His place of medical training is unknown. He married Georgia Eunice Maxey (1881–1975) in 1906; they had three children. He died of angina pectoris at the age of sixty years.

40. "Minutes of the Meetings of the State Board of Health, January 24, 1913," State Board of Health of Missouri, *Thirty-First Annual Report of the State Board of Health and Bureau of Vital Statistics of Missouri 1913* (Jefferson City, MO: Hugh Stephens Printing Company, 1913), 12–14.

41. "The Weather—Fair and Warmer," *Kansas City Star*, January 14, 1913, 1; "The Weather—Fair," *Kansas City Star*, January 26, 1912, 1; and "The Weather Colder," *Kansas City Star*, January 30, 1913, 1.

42. Wade Hampton Frost, "Epidemic Cerebrospinal Meningitis: A Review of Its Etiology, Transmission, and Specific Therapy, with Reference to Public Measures for Its Control," *Public Health Reports* 27 no. 4 (January 26, 1912): 97–112.

43. Wade Hampton Frost, "Anti-meningitis Vaccination," *Public Health Reports* 28, no. 6 (February 7, 1913): 252–54.

44. "Marvels of a Marvellous [*sic*] Winter," *Kansas City Star*, February 2, 1913, 13.

45. Arthur Hawley Parmelee, "Epidemic Cerebrospinal Meningitis," *Journal of the American Medical Association* 60, no. 9 (March 1, 1913): 659–661.

46. Simon Pendleton Kramer (1868–1940) was born in Cincinnati, Hamilton County, Ohio, as the eldest of the five children of Jacob Kramer (1839–1898), a real estate agent, and Emma Bloom (1848–1914). Simon Kramer earned his medical diploma from the Ohio Medical College in Cincinnati in 1888, worked several years as an intern at the Cincinnati City Hospital, studied abroad in London and other cities, and returned to Cincinnati to open a general practice. He served as a surgeon in the Spanish American War and as a major in the United States Army Medical Corps during World War I (July 28, 1918, to November 30, 1918). He died at the age of seventy-two years at the Marine Hospital in Baltimore, Maryland, while performing experimental work at the National Institute of Public Health. Dr. Kramer married Minnie Halle (1866–1940) in 1912; they had two children. See "Renowned Fort Thomas Scientist Dies; Dr. Simon Kramer Also Noted Surgeon," *Cincinnati Enquirer* (Cincinnati, OH), April 13, 1940, 1–2; Simon Pendleton Kramer and Rubert Boyce, "The Nature of Vaccine Immunity," *British Medical Journal* 2, no. 1714 (November 4, 1893): 989–90.

47. Tricresol is a germicidal disinfectant derived from coal tar, a thick black liquid produced by the destructive distillation of bituminous coal. Coal tar contains benzene, naphthalene, phenols (cresol), aniline, and many other organic chemicals. See E. A. Cooper, "On the Relations of Phenol and Meta-Cresol to Proteins; Contribution to Our Knowledge of the Mechanism of Disinfection," *Biochemistry Journal* 6, no. 4 (1912): 362–87; and "Tricresol," *Medical Dictionary*,

Free Dictionary, accessed June 3, 2018, http://medical-dictionary. thefreedictionary.com/tricresol.

48. "Public Opinion," *Bridgeport Times and Evening Farmer* (Bridgeport, CT), May 20, 1913, 6; and Simon Pendleton Kramer, "A Possible Source of Danger in the Use of Antimeningitis Serum," *Journal of the American Medical Association* 60, no. 18 (May 3, 1913): 1348–51.

49. Dr. Kramer wrote, "In certain of the instances reported by Dr. Kramer and Dr. Parmelee, a severe reaction followed, not on the first, but on the second or third injection of the serum, given at brief intervals. In these instances, anaphylactic shock can be excluded. Dr. Parmelee kindly supplied me with a brief account of the case from which I derive this conclusion." See Simon Flexner, "Accidents Following the Subdural Injection of the Antimeningitis Serum," *Journal of the American Medical Association* 60, no. 25 (June 21, 1913): 1939.

50. For example, "Five Deaths Are Attributed to Serum," *Evening News* (Wilkes-Barre, PA), March 19, 1913, 12; "Investigate Deaths," *Topeka State Journal*, March 19, 1913, 6; "Flexner Serum Takes Life Instead of Curing," *Grand Rapids Press* (Grand Rapids, MI), March 21, 1913, 1; and "Dangers of Anti-Meningitis Serum," *Times* (Shreveport, LA), August 16, 1914, 33.

51. Simon Flexner, "Accidents Following the Subdural Injection of the Antimeningitis Serum," *Journal of the American Medical Association* 60, no. 25 (June 21, 1913): 1937–40; and John Auer, "The Functional Effect of Experimental Intraspinal Injections with and without Preservatives," *Journal of Experimental Medicine* 21, no. 1 (January 1, 1915): 43–83. See also "Flexner Defends Serum; Discoverer and Dr. Park Deny Tricresol Caused Deaths; Disbelieve Kramer Talk; Head of Health Department Laboratories Doubts Cincinnati Story," *New York Tribune*, March 22, 1913, 2; "Flexner Defends Meningitis Cure; Rockefeller Investigator Replies to Doctor Who Said It Killed Babies; A Cincinnati Doubter; Belief That Some One [*sic*] Blundered in Using Remedy in Hospital," *Sun*, March 22, 1913, 8; "Dr. Flexner Replies; His Serum Not Cause of Death, as Cincinnati Physician Charged," *New York Times*, March 22, 1913, 10; "Hornet Nest; Stirred by Cincinnatian; Serum Discoverer Defends Remedy against Dr. Kramer's Attack; Another Queen City Physician Upholds Meningitis Treatment, Said to Be Fatal to Children," *Cincinnati Enquirer*, March 22, 1913, 14; "Flexner

Defends Serum Attacked by Kramer," *Topeka Daily Capital*, March 22, 1913, 10; and "Flexner Raps Kramer for Fling at Serum," *Cleveland Leader* (Cleveland, OH), March 22, 1913, 1.

52. Josephine B. Neal and Harry L. Abramson, "A Comparison of Tricresol and Chloroform as a Preservative in Antimeningitis Serum," *Journal of the American Medical Association* 68, no. 14 (April 7, 1917): 1935–1937.

53. "The Weather and the Crops—Considerable Precipitation and a Drop in Temperature Last Week," *Kansas City Star*, March 23, 1913, 3; and "The Weather—Snow, Colder," *Kansas City Star*, March 26, 1913, 1.

54. "A Smallpox Victim Complains; City's Contagious Hospital Sent a Woman to Negro Institution," *Kansas City Star*, March 28, 1913, 4.

55. "Keep Your Mind Off This! The Meningitis Scare Is Groundless, Doctor Castelaw Says," *Kansas City Star*, March 21, 1913, 1.

56. "High School Boy near Death; Meningitis Attacks Marion Roe, a Westport Pupil," *Kansas City Star*, April 3, 1913, 3.

57. "Planting Corn in Missouri," *Kansas City Star*, April 19, 1913, 3.

58. Abraham Sophian, *Epidemic Cerebrospinal Meningitis* (St. Louis, MO: C. V. Mosby, 1913).

59. "Medical News," *Medical Herald* 32, no. 4 (April 1913): 163.

60. "Missouri Biologic Laboratory," *Journal of the Missouri State Medical Association* 9, no. 10 (April 1913): 345.

61. Kansas City annexed the Waldo area in phases spanning a number of years. By 1909, Kansas City extended its southern boundary from Forty-Ninth Street to Seventy-Seventh Street, which included a portion of Waldo. The Sophian-Hall-Alexander Biologic Company's serum farm was located at Eighty-Seventh Street and Wornall Road. See LaDene Morton, *The Waldo Story: The Home of Friendly Merchants* (Charleston, SC: History Press, 2012), 55, 58; and "To Battle Meningitis: Farm Is to Prevent Shortage in Necessary Serum," *Fort Wayne Sentinel*, August 24, 1912, 13.

62. The American Medical Association created the Council on Pharmacy and Chemistry in the spring of 1905 to study new medicines advertised to physicians and publish the results of these investigations in the *Journal of the American Medical Association* under the title of "New and Nonofficial Remedies." Originally, twelve physicians divided into committees on chemistry, pharmacy, and pharmacology to perform the investigations. See J. H. Long, "On the Work of

the Council on Pharmacy and Chemistry of the American Medical Association," *Science* 32, no. 834 (December 23, 1910): 889–901.

63. "New and Nonofficial Remedies," *Journal of the American Medical Association* 60, no. 14 (April 5, 1913): 1074.

64. Rush English Castelaw, "Cerebrospinal Meningitis," Hospital and Health Board, *Fifth Annual Report of the Hospital and Health Board of Kansas City, Missouri, for Fiscal Year April 16, 1912, to April 21, 1913, Inclusive* (1913), 30.

65. Dr. Wheeler continued, "I kept the sanitary inspectors at work in this district most of the fall [1912] and early winter months [1913], urging that all places where many people were classed together should be cleaned with water and soap and disinfectant, such as formaldehyde and a hot soda solution; painting and whitewashing all establishments used as rooming houses; and to require all rooming houses to have bathtubs. This I believe had to do somewhat with reducing the number of people stricken with meningitis, for it is not one-third the number that we had the previous year [1912]. Cerebrospinal fever usually follows a long drought and as this year has been a rainless season throughout the country, I am quite uneasy for fear of a return of this disease this fall and winter [1913–1914]." "Cerebrospinal Meningitis," Hospital and Health Board, *Fifth Annual Report of the Hospital and Health Board of Kansas City, Missouri, for Fiscal Year April 16, 1912, to April 21, 1913, Inclusive* (Kansas City, MO: Hospital and Health Board, 1913), 56–57.

66. Hospital and Health Board, "Contagious and Infectious Diseases," *Sixth Annual Report of the Hospital and Health Board of Kansas City, Missouri, for Fiscal Year April 21, 1913, to April 20, 1914, Inclusive* (Kansas City, MO: Hospital and Health Board, 1914), 87.

67. "The Weather Was Unsettled," *Kansas City Star*, May 9, 1913, 1.

68. "Significant Weather Events of the Century for Missouri," Missouri Climate Center, University of Missouri College of Agriculture, Food, and Natural Resources, accessed May 30, 2018, http://climate.missouri.edu/sigwxmo.php.

69. "Book Reviews," *Cleveland Medical Journal* 12, no. 8 (August 1913): 573; and "Book Reviews," *Northwest Medicine* (Portland, OR; Seattle, WA; and Boise, ID) 5, no. 8 (August 1913): 237.

70. "The Doctor's Library," *Medical Herald* 32, no. 6 (June 1913): 229.

71. "Epidemic Cerebrospinal Meningitis," *American Journal of Public Health* 3, no. 12 (December 1913): 1364.

72. "Biological Products: Establishments Licensed for the Propagation and Sale of Viruses, Serums, Toxins, and Analogous Products," *Public Health Reports* 28, no. 28 (July 11, 1913): 1447.

73. "One City Hospital Empty; There Are No Patients for the Isolation Addition; Until Cooler Weather Brings on Contagious Ailments Again, the Recently Finished Building Probably Will Remain Unused," *Kansas City Star*, July 10, 1913, 2.

74. "Back to Normal This Week," *Kansas City Star*, August 17, 1913, 1.

CHAPTER 7

THE EPIDEMIC ENDS, 1913-1914

D uring the summer of 1913, health department officials and private physicians in Kansas City wondered about a return of the cerebrospinal meningitis epidemic during the upcoming cold months of late 1913 and the first half of 1914. Dr. Wheeler, for one, remained fearful.[1] However, a review of the epidemic's behavior during the cold months of 1910–1911, 1911–1912, and 1912–1913 showed a prevalence curve characteristic of the disease and favorable for a light load of the disease in Kansas City during the cold months of late 1913 and the first half of 1914. Recall that the prevalence of cerebrospinal meningitis in Kansas City was so low for more than a decade (1900–1910) that the Kansas City health department officials left its monitoring to the local newspapers. From May 1911 through December 1911, its prevalence was measured at *1.6 cerebrospinal meningitis cases per 10,000 Kansas City residents*, as previously noted. From January 1912 to July 1912, the prevalence of cerebrospinal meningitis spiked to *16.6 cerebrospinal meningitis cases per 10,000 Kansas City residents*, also as noted earlier.[2] The prevalence of the disease then slackened during the cold months of late 1912 and early 1913 to *4.8 cerebrospinal meningitis cases per 10,000 Kansas City residents*.[3]

By comparison, the New York City (Manhattan and the Bronx) cerebrospinal meningitis epidemic prevalences during the cold months of 1894 through 1907 showed a similar curve. The prevalences of cerebrospinal meningitis cases in New York City were low from 1894 through 1903. In 1904, the cerebrospinal meningitis prevalence rose to *4.6 cerebrospinal meningitis cases per 10,000 New York City residents*. In 1905, the prevalence increased further to *6.3 cerebrospinal meningitis cases per 10,000 New York City residents*. In 1906 and in 1907, the prevalences fell to *2.5* and *1.8 cerebrospinal meningitis cases per 10,000 New York City residents*, respectively.[4]

If the behavior of the Kansas City cerebrospinal meningitis epidemic in 1913–1914 followed the New York City curve, its prevalence likely would fall below a prevalence of *4.8 cerebrospinal meningitis cases per 10,000 Kansas City residents*, even reaching pre-epidemic prevalence levels. Dr. Wheeler remained cautious, however, saying, "Cerebrospinal fever usually follows a long drought and as this year has been a rainless season throughout the country, I am quite uneasy for fear of a return of this disease this fall and winter [1913–1914]."[1]

Other people were not so concerned with the return of the disease. For example, on Monday, July 14, 1913, Mrs. Catherine Beebe Cross Barnes,[5] the forty-seven-year-old owner of a property near the Sophian-Hall-Alexander Biologic Company's serum farm, wrote a letter to the editor of the *Kansas City Star*. The letter, reprinted below, was titled "Serum Farm a Menace? A Property Owner Protests against Germ Inoculation in the City."[6]

> *To The Star*: As an adjoining property owner to the Sophian-Hall-Alexander serum farm at the southwest corner of Seventy-Third and Main Streets, I wish to say that the property owners in the vicinity have been protesting since last January against this farm being conducted within the city limits and in one of the largest school districts in the city. We believe this to be a dangerous nuisance to the health of the public.

A large barn for the accommodation of at least twelve horses was built. From this barn, a sewer was built to within a few feet of the north line of this tract of land from which the sewage from this barn flows directly into the natural stream of running water on the Badger tract, then into the stream a few feet north on my property, and so on along the line into other property. My stock, as well as all the other people's stock along the line is obliged to drink this water.

The drainage from this barn contains the water used in the inoculation and dressing the wounds of these horses and incidentally any germs the doctors may drop in the process of inoculation.

The city is compelling the dairymen to give their cows pure water, while refusing to have this farm move outside of the city limits, it is virtually forcing our stock to drink water contaminated by germs of meningitis, diphtheria and perhaps other diseases. While these pathologists maintain there is no danger of contagion, yet they say if an animal has an open cut and comes in direct contact with one of these animals it might contract the disease. There is just a wire fence between their tract and mine.

While we all know that this and similar places have to be maintained for the benefit of science, their proper place is outside the city limits.

These doctors claim there is no suffering, but if one is to judge from appearances it would be a difficult task to convince a person that they do not suffer.

These doctors claim also that the horses do not die. All the neighbors can testify that five dead horses have been taken from there since last November [1912]; two of them in one week.

When I put this matter before the board of health I was advised to move! Is all of Waldo going to be obliged to move in order to give full sway to these pathologists to create germs within the city limits?

Hasn't Kansas City with its one-quarter million inhabitants the power to rid itself of this nuisance planted right in the center of one of the residence districts of the city?

Catherine C. Barnes, 7246 Main Street[6]

When she received no response to her letter, Mrs. Barnes sent a second letter to the editor, which the *Kansas City Star* published eleven days later, on Friday, July 25, 1913. Titled "Germs on Wornall Road: Horses Inoculated with Meningitis a Terror to South Side Residents,"[7] it read,

To The Star: What is the good of swatting the fly[8] when things like this are going on?

The horses from the Sophian-Hall-Alexander serum farm at the southwest corner of Seventy-Third and Main streets are driven through the south end of the city every week.

After being inoculated with meningitis and diphtheria germs these horses with the blood dripping from them, are taken from this farm to a pasture in the vicinity of Eighty-First Street and Wornall Road.

At a committee meeting of the city council held on January 31, 1913, at the request of the protesting property owners, these doctors promised to take these horses away without further trouble. True, they did take them away on April 29 [1913] for a week!

They have been brought back and forth on the most prominent public highway—the Wornall Road—in Jackson county [*sic*] once a week.

Think of the millions of germs that the hundreds of motorists who travel this road daily have spread through the air in the whole surrounding country. And yet the board of health doesn't see fit to declare the serum farm a nuisance. It is becoming a terror to the neighborhood.

They took another dead horse away from this farm Thursday, July 10 [1913].

Catherine Cross Barnes, 7246 Main Street[7]

The Sophian-Hall-Alexander Laboratory responded with a letter to the editor of the *Kansas City Star* that appeared on Sunday, July 27, 1913. The title of the letter was "Serum Farm Owners Explain, No Danger of Infection from Horses, the Proprietors Say."[9] The letter read,

To The Star: We have just learned that some people in the neighborhood of our antitoxin farm at Wornall Road and Seventy-First Street, through ignorance of the facts, have been unduly alarmed about our antitoxin farm; and we must believe unintentionally by spreading incorrect reports, have been causing unrest and uneasiness in the neighborhood.

Our antitoxin farm has passed the United States government inspection for the production of the various sera and antitoxins. The federal license is granted when the premises, upon which these products are produced, are absolutely sanitary and furthermore that they must be no menace to the people who live on the grounds or in the vicinity.

We have caretakers living on the grounds, and no time have they suffered from any infections or any diseases that might possibly be traced to the horses. Our ruffled neighbor, so far as we know, has also been blessed with the best of health. The farm has also passed the inspection and approval of the Kansas City board of health.

The horses that are kept on this farm are used for medicinal purposes; not to cause disease, but to cure disease. Our horses are used for the production of such serums and antitoxins as will cure diphtheria, lockjaw, meningitis, blood poisoning, and other similar diseases. The horses are not suffering from these diseases. If they were it would be a serious menace to use their serum medicinally.

These horses are injected with the dead and destroyed germs that produce different diseases. This material that is used to inject the horses cannot produce the diseases for which we attempt to produce curative serums. The horses are healthy; eat, look, and act like any other horses, except, of course, for a period of one day when they are injected, when sometimes they are depressed and the site of injection is sore.

We cannot understand the statement which appeared to the effect that these horses walk around dripping blood. This is an absolute untruth. We must believe the person who made this statement saw red at the time they so stated. To a casual observer these horses are no different than any other horses.

We are very anxious to do everything possible to safeguard the public and have done everything in this respect. Furthermore, we feel that the judgment and licenses granted by the highest authorities, United States government and Kansas City board of health, must be accepted as to the inoculous [sic] character of these horses.

Sophian-Hall-Alexander Lab[9]

There were no further letters to the newspaper from either Mrs. Barnes or the Sophian-Hall-Alexander Biologic Company. The altercation might have faded because Dr. Sophian already was in New York City negotiating the sale of the Sophian-Hall-Alexander Biologic Company to Mr. Theodore Weicker[10] and Mr. Lowell Mason Palmer,[11] owners of the Brooklyn-based pharmaceutical company E. R. Squibb[12] and Sons (founded in 1858). After acquiring the company in 1905, both owners had worked to extend the line of the company's products and produce larger quantities of materials already sold by the company.[13] In July 1913, the only biologics produced and sold by E. R. Squibb and Sons were bacterial cultures and culture media.[14] It is unknown how or when Dr. Sophian first came into contact with Mr. Weicker and Mr. Mason to discuss the possible acquisition. If the purchase was realized, the assets of the Sophian-Hall-Alexander Biologic Company were to be transferred to New Jersey.

Meanwhile, in August 1913, there were no new cases of cerebrospinal meningitis or deaths from the disease in Kansas City, according to the Hospital and Health Board.[15] The weather was so hot it had killed forty-nine people. Dr. Wheeler said, "It's the hot weather picking off the weakest. In only one or two cases in today's list is heat the direct cause of death."[16]

In mid-September 1913, E. R. Squibb and Sons acquired the Sophian-Hall-Alexander Biologic Company for an unknown price. Furthermore, the company hired Dr. Sophian to design and direct the company's new research division located near the Raritan River in New Brunswick, Middlesex County, New Jersey.[17, 18] Dr. Hall submitted the following letter to the *Medical Herald* to explain the reason for the departure from Kansas City of the Sophian-Hall-Alexander Biologic Company:

> Four years ago, the need of a laboratory in Kansas City for Pasteur and Wassermann work brought into existence the American Biologic Company, which Dr. Nesbit was brought here by me to become director, and for three years very satisfactory work was done. The widespread epidemic of meningitis during 1912 led me to enlarge this laboratory to produce meningitis and other sera; Dr. Sophian, an expert from the New York Research, was installed as director of the enlarged Sophian-Hall-Alexander Laboratory. Experience soon showed that a larger commercial concern must needs handle an extensive serum business, so a few weeks ago this serum company was sold to the Squibbs Company to be made part of their great pharmaceutical establishment in the east; thus, the Sophian-Hall-Alexander Biologic Company passed into history by absorption.
>
> The necessity for Pasteur and Wassermann work in Kansas City is vastly more apparent now than ever before, and to fill this need I will open a new laboratory for this work on October 1st, 1913, in connection with my clinical pathologic work,

at 1208 Wyandotte street [the site of the former
Sophian-Hall-Alexander Laboratory], where I hope
to welcome you, and serve you in the future.[17]

Dr. Sophian's reasons for selling the company have been lost
to history. On Sunday, September 28, 1913, within days of the
sale of the Sophian-Hall-Alexander Biologic Company to E. R.
Squibb and Sons, Dr. Sophian and his wife, Estelle, welcomed their
firstborn child at the New York Medical College and Hospital for
Women in New York City.[19] They named their daughter Emily
Sophian.[20]

On Monday, September 29, 1913, four carloads of horses
from the Sophian-Hall-Alexander Biologic Company serum
farm in Kansas City reached New Brunswick, New Jersey. They
were stabled in a privately owned barn in New Brunswick until
completion of the new barn designed by Dr. Sophian and built by
E. R. Squibb Research and Biological Laboratories. Meanwhile,
Dr. Sophian leased a suite of offices in the Bartle Building on
Church Street, New Brunswick, New Jersey.[21]

On October 11, 1913, the *Journal of the American Medical
Association* published a transfer of agency for the Sophian-Hall-
Alexander Laboratories. The journal item read, "The biologic
products formerly manufactured by the Sophian-Hall-Alexander
Laboratories, Kansas City, Mo. (described in *The Journal*, AMA,
April 5, 1913, p. 1074, and April 19, 1913, p. 1227, Sept. 6, 1913,
p. 771) are now manufactured and sold by E. R. Squibb and Sons,
New York."[22]

In December 1913, Mr. Alexander joined Dr. Sophian in New
Brunswick, New Jersey, as a serum chemist at the newly named E.
R. Squibb Research and Biological Laboratories.[23] Mr. Deaken and
his family apparently returned to New York City sometime after
the birth of his daughter Marion in Missouri in 1914.

On Thursday, January 1, 1914, the State Board of Health of
Missouri's new officers voted to discontinue its "contract with the
Sophian-Hall-Alexander Chemical [sic] Company, by returning all
vaccines to the company that the office ... had on hand and thereafter

cease to deal in antitoxins." The board opted to secure the state's "antirabic serum from the Surgeon General, USA, as promised by him free of charge, and treat any cases of rabies that may come to this office [in Jefferson City, Cole County, Missouri] for the same."[24] This change could not have been good news for Dr. Hall.

The aggregated data collected by the Hospital and Health Board from mid-April 1913 to mid-April 1914 showed a total of thirty-nine cases of cerebrospinal meningitis and twenty-seven deaths.[15] Thus, the Kansas City cerebrospinal meningitis prevalence for the aforementioned twelve months was *1.56 cerebrospinal meningitis cases per 10,000 Kansas City residents*. The Kansas City cerebrospinal meningitis epidemic of 1911–1913 was over.

Of the thirty-nine individuals with cerebrospinal meningitis in Kansas City between mid-April 1913 and mid-April 1914, fourteen had received their care in the Kansas City General Hospital. Of the fourteen, six died (a mortality rate of 43 percent), five were well after their infection, and three were improved.[25]

On Tuesday, June 2, 1914, Dr. Castelaw resigned as the superintendent of the Kansas City General Hospital. He told the Hospital and Health Board, "I am not a kicker. My record shows nothing against me and I am willing to let it stand for me. There has always been an influence in the hospital itself which has made good hospital administration impossible. I have never known of a place where it required so much energy to produce so little results."[26] The new members of the Hospital and Health Board,[27] appointed by Mayor Henry Lee Jost,[28] had requested Dr. Castelaw's resignation, but they refused to discuss it further. Two of the three members[26] said that they had not requested his resignation. An unnamed source who had held an official position in the hospital for six or seven years remarked, "The trouble started when the previous hospital and health board resigned. The new board has always thought it should have its 'own man.' The thing is entirely political."[26] The new man was not so new; he was Dr. George P. Pipkin, who took charge of the Kansas City General Hospital on July 1, 1914, while also continuing his duties as head of the Old Hospital.[29]

CHAPTER 7 NOTES

1. "Cerebrospinal Meningitis," Hospital and Health Board, *Fifth Annual Report of the Hospital and Health Board of Kansas City, Missouri, for Fiscal Year April 16, 1912, to April 21, 1913, Inclusive* (1913), 56–57.

2. "Report on Meningitis," Hospital and Health Board, *Fourth Annual Report of the Hospital and Health Board of Kansas City, Missouri, for Fiscal Year April 17, 1911, to April 15, 1912, Inclusive* (Kansas City, MO: Hospital and Health Board, 1912), 103.

3. Hospital and Health Board, *Fourth Annual Report of the Hospital and Health Board of Kansas City, Missouri, for Fiscal Year April 17, 1911, to April 15, 1912, Inclusive* (Kansas City, MO: Hospital and Health Board, 1912), 106.

4. Charles F. Bolduan, "Cerebrospinal Meningitis from the Standpoint of Public Health," *Medical Times* 36, no. 7 (July 1908): 193.

5. Catherine (Kate) Beebe Cross Barnes (1866–1924) was born in Kansas City as one of the five children of Asa Beebe Cross (1826–1894), a Kansas City architect, and Rachel Genevieve Taylor (1838–1890), a young widow with a small son, William E. Taylor (1856–1883). In 1891, twenty-five-year-old Catherine Cross married twenty-two-year-old Alfred Edward Barnes (1869–1928), an English-born construction specialist who assisted his father-in-law in building the Jackson County Courthouse in 1888. Catherine and Alfred Barnes had two sons, Alfred E. Barnes Jr. (1892–1960) and Asa Beebe Cross Barnes (1894–1991); both became architects. Catherine and Alfred E. Barnes Sr. divorced. Alfred Sr. moved to Texas to continue his construction career, remarried in 1901, and had three more children. Catherine Barnes remained in Kansas City, did not remarry, and raised her two sons, both of whom lived with her at 7246 Main Street, Kansas City, until her death in 1924 from kidney failure and diabetes mellitus at the age of fifty-seven years. "Asa Beebe Cross (1826–1894) Papers," State Historical Society of Missouri Research Center-Kansas City, State Historical Society of Missouri, accessed May 3, 2018, https://shsmo.org/manuscripts/kansascity/k0082.pdf; and "Mrs. Catherine C. Barnes Dies; End Comes to Daughter of Early Day Architect Here," *Kansas City Star*, March 30, 1924, 8.

6. "Serum Farm a Menace? A Property Owner Protests against German Inoculation in the City," *Kansas City Star*, July 14, 1913, 4.

7. "Germs on Wornall Road; Horses Inoculated with Meningitis a Terror to South Side Residents," *Kansas City Star*, July 25, 1913, 2.

8. Public health authorities of this era condemned the common house fly because it deposited germs on food. Sanitary experts pointed out that the fly bred in the filth of barnyards and city dumps; it possessed twelve thousand foot hairs that exuded a slimy fluid; and its hairy legs could carry one hundred thousand bacteria. Health authorities encouraged people to "Swat the fly!" with a flyswatter, which was named by Dr. Samuel Jay Crumbine (1862–1954), the longtime head of the Kansas State Board of Health. See "House Fly Catechism," *Bulletin of the Kansas State Board of Health* 7, no. 4 (April 1911): 75–76, 80.

9. "Serum Farm Owners Explain; No Danger of Infection from Horses, the Proprietors Say," *Kansas City Star*, July 27, 1913, 2.

10. Johann Adam Theodor (Theodore) Wilhelm Weicker (1861–1940) was born in Darmstadt, Hessen, Germany, as the eldest of the four children of Ludwig Christian Weicker (1839–1897) and Anna Marie Elisabeth Momberger (1841–1925). He received his early formal education in Darmstadt and joined E. (Emanuel) Merck, the German drug manufacturer. He moved to New York City in 1887 to open a Merck branch office. Between 1887 and 1891, he earned degrees in pharmacy and pharmaceutical chemistry at the College of Pharmacy of Columbia University, and he became a naturalized citizen of the United States in 1890. While he was studying at the College of Pharmacy, he became interested in the work of Dr. Edward Robinson Squibb (see note 12 below). In 1891, George Friedrich Merck (1867–1926), a member of the Merck family in Darmstadt, moved to New York City to oversee the Merck branch office. Soon after settling in New York City, Mr. Merck cofounded Merck and Company with Theodore Weicker. In the beginning, the company concentrated on the importation of drugs and chemicals primarily from the parent company, E. Merck. In 1903, Theodore Weicker surprised the industry by selling his share of the business to George Merck. He used his capital to copurchase with Lowell Mason Palmer E. R. Squibb and Sons, a business that then consisted of one bookkeeper, one salesman, and one hundred laboratory employees. He and Mr. Palmer built the organization into one of the largest drug firms in the world. He married Florence Edith Palmer (the daughter of Lowell Mason Palmer) in 1901; they had four children. Theodore Weicker died in 1940 at the age of eighty. See Leon Gortler, "Merck in

America: The First 70 Years from Fine Chemicals to Pharmaceutical Giant," *Bulletin for the History of Chemistry* 25, no.1 (2000): 1–9; "Theodore Weicker Dies; Dr. E. R. Squibb Executive," *Brooklyn Daily Eagle*, August 7, 1940, 13; "Theodore Weicker Dies in New York; Realized Life-long Dream at Opening of Research Institute Here," *Central New Jersey Home News*, August 7, 1940, 1; "Big Chemical Company Has Been Reorganized; E. R. Squibb and Sons, with Increased Capital, Will Enlarge Work in Brooklyn; Founder a Famous Chemist; For Nearly Half a Century He Conducted Business Here with His Sons," *Brooklyn Daily Eagle*, February 1, 1905, 5; J. L. Sturchio, ed., *Values and Visions: A Merck Century* (Rahway, NJ: Merck and Company, 1991); and William Haynes, ed., *American Chemical Industry: The Chemical Companies* (New York: D. Van Nostrand Company, 1949).

11. Lowell Mason Palmer (1845–1915) was born in Chester Center, Geauga County, Ohio, as one of the six children of Chester Urban Palmer (1812–1894), a farmer, and Achsah Melvin (1810–1850). He served throughout the four years of the American Civil War, commanding a battery at the age of seventeen years. He was discharged at the rank of captain. He moved to Brooklyn, New York City, and founded the Palmer Dock Company in the Eastern District of Brooklyn, and for many years, he served as its president. He next founded the Brooklyn Cooperage Company, which made the large quantities of barrels used by the American Sugar Refining Company. In 1874, he brought the first railroad to Brooklyn, and he also built the first elevated coal pockets in the old City of Brooklyn. After retiring from all of these companies, he served as a director of many companies. In 1905, at the age of sixty, he purchased E. R. Squibb and Sons with Theodore Weicker. He married Harriet Miriam Wilde (1847–1876) in 1869; they had no children. He married Grace Humphrey Foote (1854–1919) in 1877; they had eight children. "Lowell M. Palmer Dies at Stamford; Founder of the Palmer Dock Company and Brooklyn Cooperage Company; Director of Academy of Music; Mr. Palmer Had a Long and Notable Career in Big Business Enterprises in Brooklyn," *Brooklyn Daily Eagle* (New York City, NY), September 30, 1915, 1.

12. Dr. Edward Robinson Squibb (1819–1900), a Quaker physician-chemist, founded the Squibb Chemical and Pharmaceutical Laboratories in 1858 in Brooklyn to manufacture and sell high-quality ether, chloroform, and other chemical medicinal agents

to the United States government and other customers. Dr. E. R. Squibb was born in Wilmington, Delaware, as the eldest of the five children of James Robinson Squibb (1796–1852) and Catherine Harrison Bonsall (1798–1833). Dr. E. R. Squibb's three sisters died from typhoid fever in 1831, his mother died of typhoid fever in 1833, his father died in 1852, and his brother died serving in the Civil War in 1862. E. R. Squibb earned his medical degree from the Thomas Jefferson Medical College in Philadelphia, Pennsylvania, in 1845; oversaw the medical station at the Brooklyn Navy Yard as an assistant surgeon in the United States Navy; and opened his own laboratory in 1857. When the Civil War broke out, the government used Dr. E. R. Squibb's skill in the preparation of pharmaceutical supplies to good account. Dr. E. R. Squibb married Caroline Lownds Cook (1833–1905) in 1852; they had four children. When Dr. E. R. Squibb died in 1900, his two sons, Dr. Edward Hamilton Squibb and Charles Fellows Squibb (a third son died in childhood), ran the company until 1905, when they sold the company to Theodore Weicker, who became the company president, and Lowell Mason Powell. See "Dr. Edward R. Squibb," *New York Times*, October 27, 1900, 7; "Squibb, Edward Robinson," Reynolds-Finley Historical Library, University of Alabama at Birmingham, accessed September 23, 2017, https://library.uab.edu/locations/reynolds/collections/civil-war/medical-figures/edward-robinson-squibb; Lawrence G. Blochman, *Doctor Squibb: The Life and Times of a Rugged Idealist* (New York: Simon and Schuster, 1958); and William A. McGarry, *The Story of the House of Squibb* (New York: Doubleday, Doran, and Company, 1931).

13. "Big Chemical Company Has Been Reorganized; E. R. Squibb and Sons, with Increased Capital, Will Enlarge Work in Brooklyn; Founder a Famous Chemist; For Nearly Half a Century He Conducted Business Here with His Sons," *Brooklyn Daily Eagle*, February 1, 1905, 5; "Architect Tells Plans of New Industry; Factories Here to be Larger Than Those in Brooklyn, Where 2,000 Hands Are Employed," *Daily Home News* (New Brunswick, NJ), November 25, 1905, 1.

14. "Bacteriological Products," *Squibb's Materia Medica, 1906 Edition, Part II* (New York: J. R. Taplay Company, 1906), 343, 347.

15. Hospital and Health Board, "Contagious and Infectious Diseases," *Sixth Annual Report of the Hospital and Health Board of Kansas*

City, Missouri, for Fiscal Year April 21, 1913, to April 20, 1914, Inclusive (Kansas City, MO: Hospital and Health Board, 1914), 140.

16. "Death in Hot Wave; Forty-One Named on List," *Kansas City Star*, August 11, 1913, 1.

17. Frank J. Hall, "Correspondence: Laboratory of Clinical Pathology," *Medical Herald* 32, no. 11 (November 1913), 431.

18. A history of the Squibb Company is beyond the scope of this book. A rough outline of its activities between 1906 and 1913 is available in the following newspaper articles: "Squibb Concern Will Come Here," *Central New Jersey Home News* (New Brunswick, NJ), June 2, 1906, 1; "Squibb Concern Takes Steps to Enlarge Plant; New Buildings Will Shortly Be Erected at Site along Raritan River Railroad—President Here Yesterday," *Central New Jersey Home News*, July 31, 1913, 1; "Squibb Plant in Operation, after 5 Years," *Central New Jersey Home News*, January 11, 1913, 1; "Laboratory to Be Built First at Squibb Plant: Work Will Be Commenced Shortly in Carrying Out Extension Plans—Steel Building 60 by 100 Feet," *Daily Home News* (New Brunswick, NJ), August 12, 1913, 1; and "New Building at Squibb Works," *Daily Home News*, August 12, 1913, 4; "Fireproof Laboratory for the Squibb Plant," *Central New Jersey Home News*, August 21, 1913, 1; "Personal," *Central New Jersey Home News*, March 3, 1914, 9; "Doctors Pay Visit to Squibb's Laboratory," *Central New Jersey Home News*, April 16, 1914, 3; "Squibb Plant Puts This City in Touch with the Big War," *Central New Jersey Home News*, October 15, 1914, 4; and "Work of Squibb Laboratories Is Explained; Dr. Sophien [*sic*] Tells How Anti-Toxins Are Produced—Output Is Used in Camps of the Warring European Nations," *Central New Jersey Home News*, October 17, 1914, 7.

19. "New York Medical College and Hospital for Women," *Journal of the American Institute of Homeopathy* 7 (July 1914–June 1915): 1223; and Sylvain Cazalet, "History of the New York Medical College and Hospital for Women," accessed September 27, 2017, http://www.homeoint.org/cazalet/histo/newyork.htm.

20. State of New York Certificate and Record of Birth for Emily Sophian, born September 28, 1913, Certificate Number 48775. Dr. Robert Tilden Frank (1875–1949), a gynecologist, obstetrician, and pioneer in endocrinology and the sex hormones, signed the birth certificate. Emily Sophian (1913–1994) was the mother and mother-in-law of the coauthors of this book.

21. "Horses for the Squibbs Arrive," *Central New Jersey Home News*, September 29, 1913, 2.

22. "Transfer of Agency," New and Nonofficial Remedies, *Journal of the American Medical Association* 61, no. 15 (October, 11, 1913): 1377. See also "Reliable Medicines," *Journal of the Missouri State Medical Association* 10, no. 5 (November 1913): 187.

23. "Just Personals," *Central New Jersey Home News*, November 25, 1913, 8.

24. "Jefferson City, Mo., Jan. 1, 1914, Minutes of the Meetings of the State Board of Health, 1914," State Board of Health of Missouri, *Thirty-Second Annual Report of the State Board of Health and Bureau of Vital Statistics of Missouri 1914* (Jefferson City, MO: Hugh Stephens Company, 1915), 8.

25. Hospital and Health Board, "Medical Diseases—General Hospital from April 21, 1913, to April 20, 1914," *Sixth Annual Report of the Hospital and Health Board of Kansas City, Missouri, for Fiscal Year April 21, 1913, to April 20, 1914, Inclusive* (Kansas City, MO: Hospital and Health Board, 1914), 122.

26. "Why Dr. Castelaw Resigned: The New Hospital Board Wanted the Job for Its 'Own' Man," *Kansas City Star*, June 3, 1914, 1.

27. The new members of the Hospital and Health Board were Thomas Martin Finn (1870–1950), president, appointed February 1, 1914; Baylis Steele (1863–1934), vice president; and John F. Wiedenmann (1871–1957), commissioner. Thomas M. Finn was in the real estate, insurance, and building businesses. Baylis Steele developed real estate and served as postmaster of Kansas City. John F. Wiedenmann owned Wiedenmann Bros. Grocery Store in Westport, Kansas. "T. M. Finn to Health Board," *Kansas City Star*, February 1, 1914, 1; "Baylis Steele Is Dead; Former Postmaster, 72 Years Old, Had Been Ill a Year; A Real Estate Operator for Years, He Developed Many Tracts in Greater Kansas City—Relative of George Washington," *Kansas City Star*, April 25, 1935, 11; and "John F. Wiedenmann, Member of Old Westport Family Was 86; Formerly He and a Brother Were Proprietors of a Grocery," *Kansas City Times*, July 26, 1957, 18.

28. Henry Lee Jost (1873–1950) served as mayor of Kansas City, Missouri (1912–1916), and as a United States congressman (1923–1925). He was born in New York City to Simeon Jost and Lena Bahr. He became orphaned at the age of six years and lived at the Five Points Mission for Homeless Children on Manhattan's Lower East Side. An orphan train took him to Hopkins, Nodaway County, Missouri, where

Judge Dale adopted him and twenty-four other foundlings. Henry Lee Jost earned his law degree from the Kansas City Law School in 1898 and worked for the Jackson County, Missouri, prosecuting attorney's office. He began his first term in office in April 1912 amid the worst days of the Kansas City meningitis epidemic of 1911 to 1913. He oversaw the erection of the Union Station (1914) and the selection of Kansas City as the Tenth Reserve Bank District of the Federal Reserve System (1914). He married Minnie Alice Hanks of Oak Grove, Missouri, in 1911; they had two children. He died after a surgical operation at the age of seventy-six years. "Preliminary Inventory, K0270 (KA0631), Henry Lee Jost (1873–1950) Papers," State Historical Society of Missouri, accessed May 30, 2018, https://shsmo.org/manuscripts/kansascity/k0270.pdf.

29. "New General Hospital Head; Dr. George Pipkin, Recently Appointed, Takes Charge Today," *Kansas City Star*, July 1, 1914, 6.

CONCLUSION

VIOLENT AND NOT IMAGINED

The Kansas City cerebrospinal meningitis epidemic of 1911 to 1913 attained a prevalence of 16.6 *cerebrospinal meningitis cases per 10,000 Kansas City residents,* ranking it a substantial epidemic among United States cerebrospinal meningitis epidemics. The meningococcus behaved in its usual manner during the epidemic, striking people wantonly and causing slow, agonal deaths that were hard on victims' families and the physicians, nurses, and orderlies who treated and cared for the patients.

Medical social behavior was in full color during the epidemic, with many Kansas City physicians and health officials repeatedly cautioning people against imagining their symptoms (recall Dr. Luscher's imaginitis). It is unclear why the health officials and physicians did this, as dismissing laypersons' honest concerns about their health almost certainly led many of them to wait too long to obtain care for fear of hearing lectures that, as Dr. E. Albert Lieberman said to Mr. Hedrick, "such a mental condition rather attracts the infection and prepares the body for receiving rather than warding off the disease nervous case." Waiting too long for care was a death sentence that almost certainly elevated the cerebrospinal meningitis mortality rate in Kansas City.

However, the struggles of Kansas City in responding to the cerebrospinal meningitis epidemic of 1911 to 1913 were in large part due to the nature of the disease itself and the toxic severity of its strike, not to any shortcomings of the city's dedicated public health officials and community of physicians. The city health department and medical community followed state-of-the-art procedures to control the epidemic, such as providing treatment with antimeningitis serum to all afflicted patients in a special meningitis ward of the Kansas City General Hospital and collecting and tabulating the morbidity and mortality data associated with the epidemic. Despite the valiant efforts of the city health authorities and the private medical community, just when they thought they had vanquished the epidemic, it hit them so hard that they reeled at the number of cases, which were exacerbated by exhaustion of all the city's antimeningitis serum supply.

It is to the credit of the Kansas City leaders, such as Mr. William Perry Motley, and institutions, such as the *Kansas City Post*, that sought help from afar (i.e., rescue antimeningitis serum supplies from the Research Laboratory, New York City Board of Health, and consultation from Dr. Sophian) to try to correct the downward spiral and steady the city. It is also to the credit of Dr. Frank J. Hall, Kansas City pathologist, who helped stem the runaway epidemic by quietly vaccinating fifty families of victims with the meningococcal vaccine originated and ardently and tirelessly promoted by Dr. Sophian. Dr. Hall's vaccination program in Kansas City during April and May 1912 might have been the first large-scale clinical trial of the vaccine in the United States. It is a shame that Dr. Hall did not document the details of his experience somewhere and that we only know about it from references to it in Dr. Sophian's writings and speeches.

BIBLIOGRAPHY

Newspapers

Abilene Daily Reflector (Abilene, KS)

Albuquerque Journal (Albuquerque, NM)

Argus-Leader (Sioux Falls, SD)

Arkansas Gazette (Little Rock, AR)

Atchison Daily Champion (Atchison, KS)

Baltimore American (Baltimore, MD)

Boston Herald (Boston, MA)

Boston Journal (Boston, MA)

Brazil Daily Times (Brazil, IN)

Bridgeport Times and Evening Farmer (Bridgeport, CT)

Brooklyn Daily Eagle (Brooklyn, NY)

Brown County World (Brown County, KS)

Central New Jersey Home News (New Brunswick, NJ)

Chicago Tribune (Chicago, IL)

Chillicothe Morning Constitution (Chillicothe, MO)

Cincinnati Enquirer (Cincinnati, OH)

Cleveland Leader (Cleveland, OH)

Columbia Record (Columbia, SC)

Corsicana Semi-Weekly Light (Corsicana, TX)

Courier-Post (Camden, NJ)

Daily Home News (New Brunswick, NJ)

Dallas Morning News (Dallas, TX)

Emporia Gazette (Emporia, KS)

Evening Missourian (Columbia, MO)

Evening News (Wilkes-Barre, PA)

Evening Star (Washington, DC)
Evening Statesman (Walla Walla, WA)
Evening World (New York City, NY)
Fort Wayne Sentinel (Fort Wayne, IN)
Fort Worth Star-Telegram (Fort Worth, TX)
Galveston Daily News (Galveston, TX)
Gazette Glove (Kansas City, KS)
Grand Rapids Press (Grand Rapids, MI)
Greensboro Daily News (Greensboro, NC)
Hartford Courant (Hartford, CT)
Houston Post (Houston, TX)
Hutchinson News (Hutchinson, KS)
Independence Daily Reporter (Independence, KS)
Joplin Globe (Joplin, MO)
Kansas City Post (Kansas City, MO)
Kansas City Star (Kansas City, MO)
Kansas City Times (Kansas City, MO)
Kansas Democrat (Oswego, KS)
Los Angeles Times (Los Angeles, CA)
Macon Chronicle (Macon, MO)
Macon Chronicle-Herald (Macon, MO)
Marshall Republican (Marshall, MO)
Moberly Monitor-Index (Moberly, MO)
Muskogee Times-Democrat (Muskogee, OK)
New York Times (New York City, NY)
New York Tribune (New York City, NY)
Olathe Mirror (Olathe, KS)
Orlando Evening Star (Orlando, FL)
Ottawa Daily Republic (Ottawa, KS)
Philadelphia Inquirer (Philadelphia, PA)
Plaindealer (Topeka, KS)
Savannah Tribune (Savannah, GA)
Sedalia Democrat (Sedalia, MO)
Sedalia Weekly Democrat (Sedalia, MO)
St. Louis Post-Dispatch (St. Louis, MO)
Sun (New York City, NY)

Times (Shreveport, LA)
Times-Democrat (New Orleans, LA)
Topeka Daily Capital (Topeka, KS)
Topeka State Journal (Topeka, KS)
Washington Bee (Washington, DC)
Weekly Gazette Globe (Kansas City, KS)
Wheeling Daily Intelligencer (Wheeling, WV)

Books

- Abbott, Alexander Crever. *The Hygiene of Transmissible Diseases*. Philadelphia, PA: W. B. Saunders, 1899.
- Aitken, William, and Meredith Clymer. *The Science and Practice of Medicine*. Philadelphia, PA: Lindsay and Blakiston, 1868.
- Alden, Ebenezer. *Early History of the Medical Profession in Norfolk County, Mass.: An Address Delivered before the Norfolk District Medical Society at Its Annual Meeting, May 10, 1853*. Boston, MA: S. K. Whipple and Company, 1853.
- *Alumni Roster of the University of Pennsylvania*. Philadelphia, PA: University of Pennsylvania General Alumni Society, 1902.
- *Annual Announcement, Baylor University School of Medicine and School of Pharmacy, Dallas, Texas, 1910–1911*. Dallas, TX: Medical Department of Baylor University, 1910.
- *Annual Catalogue and Announcement of College of Physicians and Surgeons in the City of New York, Medical Department of Columbia College*. New York: Macgowan and Slipper, 1888.
- *Appletons' Cyclopedia of American Biography, 1600–1889*. New York: D. Appleton and Company, 1888.
- Baker, Marilyn Miller. *The History of Pathology in Texas*. Austin, TX: Texas Society of Pathologists, 1996.

- Biggs, Hermann M. *Brief History of the Campaign against Tuberculosis in New York City: Catalogue of the Tuberculosis Exhibit of the Department of Health, City of New York, 1908.* New York: Department of Health, 1908.
- Blochman, Lawrence G. *Doctor Squibb: The Life and Times of a Rugged Idealist.* New York: Simon and Schuster, 1958.
- Board of the Health of the State of Missouri. *Annual Report of the Board of Health of the State of Missouri for 1891.* Jefferson City, MO: Tribune Printing Company, 1892.
- Bone, D. M. *Kansas City Annual, 1907.* Kansas City, MO: Bishop Press, 1906.
- Bosanquet, William Cecil, and John William Henry Eyre. *Serum, Vaccines, and Toxines [sic] in Treatment and Diagnosis.* New York: Funk and Wagnalls Company, 1910.
- Brock, Thomas D. *Robert Koch: A Life in Medicine and Bacteriology.* Berlin: Springer-Verlag, 1988.
- Brown, E. Richard. *Rockefeller Medicine Men: Medicine and Capitalism in America.* Berkeley, CA: University of California Press, 1979.
- Bushel, Arthur. *Chronology of New York City Department of Health (and Its Predecessor Agencies) 1655–1966.* New York: New York City Health Department, March 1966.
- *Cactus, University of Texas Yearbook, 1906.* Austin, TX: Von Boeckmann-Jones Company, 1906.
- Carlisle, Robert Janus. *An Account of Bellevue Hospital.* New York: Society of the Alumni of Bellevue Hospital, 1893.
- *Catalogue of the Officers and Graduates of Yale University, 1701–1910.* New Haven, CT: Tuttle, Morehouse, and Taylor, 1910.
- Chernow, Ron. *Titan: The Life of John D. Rockefeller Sr.* New York: Vintage, 1984.
- Clymer, Meredith. *Epidemic Cerebro-Spinal Meningitis.* Philadelphia, PA: Lindsay and Blakiston, 1872.

- Colebrook, Leonard. *Almroth Wright: Provocative Doctor and Thinker.* London: Whitefriars Press, 1954.
- Conard, Howard Louis. *Encyclopedia of the History of Missouri: A Compendium of History.* New York: Southern History Company, 1901.
- Cooper, Page. *The Bellevue Story.* New York: Thomas Y. Crowell Company, 1948.
- Corner, George Washington. *A History of the Rockefeller Institute, 1901–1953: Origins and Growth.* New York: Rockefeller Institute Press, 1964.
- Dalton, William J. *Life of Father Bernard Donnelly with Historical Sketches of Kansas City, St. Louis, and Independence, Missouri.* Kansas City, MO: Grimes-Joyce Printing Company, 1921.
- Daniel, Thomas M. *Wade Hampton Frost, Pioneer Epidemiologist 1880–1938: Up to the Mountain.* Rochester, NY: University of Rochester Press, 2004.
- Davis, Ellis Arthur, and Edwin H. Grobe. *New Encyclopedia of Texas.* Dallas, TX: Texas Development Bureau, 1926.
- *Directory of Teachers in the Public Schools.* New York: Board of Education of the City of New York, 1905.
- Ellis, Roy. *A Civic History of Kansas City, Missouri.* Springfield, MO: Press of Elkins-Swyers Company, 1930.
- Fairbanks, Jonathan, and Clyde Edwin Tuck. *Past and Present of Green County: Early and Recent History and Genealogical Records of Many of the Representative Citizens.* La Crosse, WI: Brookhaven Press, 2012.
- Flexner, James Thomas. *An American Saga: The Story of Helen Thomas and Simon Flexner.* New York: Fordham University Press, 1993.
- Fowler, Giles. *Deaths on Pleasant Street.* Kirksville, MO: Truman State University Press, 2009.
- Galambos, Louis. *Networks of Innovation: Vaccine Development at Merck, Sharp and Dohme, and Mulford, 1895–1995.* New York: Cambridge University Press, 1997.

- *General Catalogue of the Officers and Graduates of the University of Wisconsin, 1849–1907.* Madison, WI: University Press, 1907.
- Gorman, Barbara M., Richard D. McKinzie, and Theodore A. Wilson. *From Shamans to Specialist: A History of Medicine and Health Care in Jackson County, Missouri.* Kansas City, MO: Jackson County Medical Society, 1981.
- Gould, George M. *The Jefferson Medical College of Philadelphia, 1826–1904; A History: Benefactors, Alumni, Hospital, Etc.; Its Founders, Officers, Instructors.* New York: Lewis Publishing Company, 1904.
- Hafner, Arthur Wayne. *Directory of Deceased American Physicians, 1804–1929.* Chicago, IL: American Medical Association, c. 1993.
- *Harvard College Class of 1895 Fifth Report.* Cambridge, MA: Crimson, 1915.
- *Harvard College Class of 1895, Thirty-Fifth Anniversary Report.* Cambridge, MA: Tolman-University Press, 1930.
- *Harvard University Directory.* Cambridge, MA: Harvard University Press, 1913.
- Haynes, William. *American Chemical Industry: The Chemical Companies.* New York: D. Van Nostrand Company, 1949.
- Hill, Austin Bradford. *Principles of Medical Statistics.* London: Lancet, 1967.
- Hospital and Health Board. *Fifth Annual Report of the Hospital and Health Board of Kansas City, Missouri, for Fiscal Year April 16, 1912, to April 21, 1913, Inclusive.* Kansas City, MO: Hospital and Health Board, 1913.
- Hospital and Health Board. *First Annual Report of the Board of Hospital and Health of Kansas City, Missouri, for Fiscal Year April 20, 1908, to April 19, 1909, Inclusive.* Kansas City, MO: Kansas City Board of Hospital and Health, 1909.
- Hospital and Health Board. *Fourth Annual Report of the Hospital and Health Board of Kansas City, Missouri, for*

Fiscal Year April 17, 1911, to April 15, 1912, Inclusive.
Kansas City, MO: Hospital and Health Board, 1912.

- Hospital and Health Board. *Second Annual Report of the Board of Hospital and Health of Kansas City, Missouri, for Fiscal Year April 20, 1909, to April 19, 1910, Inclusive.* Kansas City, MO: Kansas City Board of Hospital and Health, 1910.

- Hospital and Health Board. *Sixth Annual Report of the Hospital and Health Board of Kansas City, Missouri, for Fiscal Year April 21, 1913, to April 20, 1914, Inclusive.* Kansas City, MO: Hospital and Health Board, 1914.

- Hospital and Health Board. *Third Annual Report of the Hospital and Health Board of Kansas City, Missouri, for Fiscal Year April 18, 1910, to April 17, 1911, Inclusive.* Kansas City, MO: Hospital and Health Board, 1911.

- King, Moses. *King's Handbook of New York 1892.* Boston, MA: Barnes and Noble, 1892.

- Ladwig, Craig. *The Star: The First 100 Years.* Kansas City, MO: *Kansas City Star,* 1980.

- Major, Ralph Hermon. *Classic Descriptions of Disease.* Springfield, IL: Charles C. Thomas, 1959.

- *Manual of the Normal College of the City of New York, 1894.* New York: Douglas Taylor and Company, 1894.

- Maxwell, W. J. *General Alumni Catalogue of the University of Pennsylvania, 1917.* Philadelphia, PA: Alumni Association of the University, 1917.

- McGarry, William A. *The Story of the House of Squibb.* New York: Doubleday, Doran, and Company, 1931.

- *Men of Affairs in Greater Kansas City: A Newspaper Reference Work.* Kansas City, MO: Kansas City Press Club, 1912.

- Morton, LaDene. *The Waldo Story: The Home of Friendly Merchants.* Charleston, SC: History Press, 2012.

- Moursund, Walter Henrik. *A History of Baylor University, College of Medicine, 1900–1953.* Houston, TX: Gulf Printing Company, 1956.

- *New York University Alumni Catalogue, 1833–1907, Medical Alumni: University Medical-Bellevue Hospital Medical-University and Bellevue Hospital Medical.* New York: General Alumni Society, 1908.
- *Normal College Echo, First Annual, 1896.* New York: J. S. Babcock, 1896.
- *Normal College Echo, Second Annual, 1897.* New York: J. S. Babcock, 1897.
- North, Elisha. *A Treatise on a Malignant Epidemic Commonly Called Spotted Fever.* New York: T and J. Swords, 1811.
- O'Leary, Margaret R., and Dennis S. O'Leary. *The Texas Meningitis Epidemic, 1911–1913: Origin of the Meningococcal Vaccine.* Bloomington, IN: iUniverse, 2018.
- Oliver, Wade W. *The Man Who Lived for Tomorrow: A Biography of William Hallock Park, MD.* New York: E. P. Dutton, 1941.
- Porta, Miquel. *A Dictionary of Epidemiology.* Oxford, England: Oxford University Press, 2014.
- *Proceedings of the American Pharmaceutical Association at the Forty-Fourth Annual Meeting Held at Montreal, Canada, August 1896.* Baltimore, MD: American Pharmaceutical Association, 1896.
- Quebbeman, Frances E. *Medicine in Territorial Arizona.* Phoenix, AZ: Arizona Historical Foundation, 1966.
- *Revised Statutes of the State of Missouri, 1909.* Jefferson City, MO: Hugh Stephens Printing Company, 1910.
- *Scalpel: A Year Book of the University Medical College.* Kansas City, MO: Punton-Clark Publishing Company, 1909.
- Scott, David. *Epidemic Disease in Ghana, 1901–1960.* London: Oxford University Press, 1965.
- Shakespeare, William. *The Merchant of Venice.* Cambridge, England: Cambridge University Press, 2018.

- Shrady, John. *The College of Physicians and Surgeons, New York: A History.* New York: Lewis Publishing Company, 1903.
- Siegel, Jane D., Emily Rhinehart, Marguerite Jackson, Linda Chiarella, and the Healthcare Infection Control Practices Advisory Committee. *Guideline for Isolation Precautions: Preventing Transmission of Infectious Agents in Healthcare Settings (2007).* Atlanta, GA: Centers for Disease Control and Prevention, 2007.
- Sophian, Abraham. *Epidemic Cerebrospinal Meningitis.* St. Louis, MO: C. V. Mosby Company, 1913.
- State Board of Health of Missouri. *Thirty-First Annual Report of the State Board of Health and Bureau of Vital Statistics of Missouri 1913.* Jefferson City, MO: Hugh Stephens Printing Company, 1913.
- State Board of Health of Missouri. *Thirty-Second Annual Report of the State Board of Health and Bureau of Vital Statistics of Missouri 1914.* Jefferson City, MO: Hugh Stephens Company, 1915.
- State Board of Health of Missouri. *Twenty-Ninth Annual Report of the State Board of Health of Missouri 1911.* Jefferson City, MO: Hugh Stephens Printing Company, 1911.
- Stevens, Walter Barlow. *Centennial History of Missouri, The Center State, 1821–1915.* Chicago, IL: S. J. Clarke Publishing Company, 1915–1921.
- *Supplementary History of the Yale Class of 1853.* New Haven, CT: Tuttle, Morehouse, and Taylor, 1894.
- Thayer, Alfred Edward. *Compend of Pathology: General and Special; A Student's Manual in One Volume.* Philadelphia, PA: P. Blakiston's Son and Company, 1906.
- Thayer, Alfred Edward. *Compend of Special Pathology.* Philadelphia, PA: P. Blakiston's Son and Company, 1902.
- *Thirtieth Annual Report of the Normal College for the Year Ending December 31, 1900; Catalogue of the Students*

Together with the Class Standing of Each Student. New York: Regents of the State of New York, 1900.

- *Transactions of the Section on Pathology and Physiology of the American Medical Association at the Sixty-Third Annual Session, Held at Atlantic City, NJ, June 4 to 7, 1912.* Chicago, IL: American Medical Association, 1912.
- Turpin, Rees, George King, and Charles L. Shannon. *Charter and Revised Ordinances of Kansas City, 1909.* Kansas City, MO: Frank T. Riley Publishing Company, 1909.
- *University of Wisconsin Alumni Directory, 1849–1911.* Madison, WI: University of Wisconsin, 1912.
- Valleix, François-Louis-Isidore. *Guide du Médecin Praticien or Résumé Général de Pathologie Interne et de Thérapeutique Appliqués.* Paris: Chez J.–B. Bailliere, 1844–1848.
- von Pirquet, Clemens F., and Béla Schick. *Serum Sickness.* Philadelphia, PA: Williams and Wilkins, 1951.
- Waksman, Selman. *The Brilliant and Tragic Life of W. M. W. Haffkine: Bacteriologist.* New Brunswick, NJ: Rutgers University Press, 1964.
- Weichselbaum, Anton. *The Elements of Pathological Histology.* London: Longmans, Green, and Company, 1895.
- Whitney, Carrie Westlake. *Kansas City Missouri, Its History and Its People, 1800–1908.* Chicago, IL: S. J. Clarke Publishing Company, 1908.
- Williams, Ralph Chester. *The United States Public Health Service, 1798–1950.* Washington, DC: Officers Association of the United States Public Health Service, 1951.
- Winslow, C.-E. A. *The Life of Hermann M. Biggs, Physician and Statesman of the Public Health.* Philadelphia, PA: Lea and Febiger, 1929.
- Wright, Almroth Edward. *Vaccine Therapy: Its Administration, Value, and Limitations.* London: Longmans, Green, and Company, 1910.

Professional Journals and Magazines

Alumni Magazine, Carleton College
American Journal of Clinical Pathology
American Journal of Nursing
American Journal of Public Health
American Journal of the Diseases of Children
American Journal of the Medical Sciences
Berliner Klinische Wochesnschrift
Biochemistry Journal
Boston Medical and Surgical Journal
British Medical Journal
Bulletin for the History of Chemistry
Bulletin of the Kansas State Board of Health
Canadian Journal of Comparative Medicine
Catholic Key Online News 2018
Cleveland Medical Journal
Clinical Infectious Diseases
Cold Spring Harbor Perspectives in Medicine
Crisis, A Record of the Darker Races
Deutsch Medizinische Wochenschrift
Emporia State Research Studies
Graduate Magazine of the University of Kansas
Handbook of Texas Online
Heritage of the Great Plains
Jackson County Medical Journal
Journal de Médecine, Chirurgie, Pharmacie, Etc.
Journal of Experimental Medicine
Journal of Infectious Diseases
Journal of Pathology and Bacteriology
Journal of the American Institute of Homoeopathy
Journal of the American Medical Association
Journal of the History of Medicine and Allied Sciences
Journal of the Missouri State Medical Association
Journal of the National Medical Association
Journal of the Oklahoma State Medical Association
Kansas City Medical Index-Lancet

Medical and Agricultural Register
Medical Herald
Medical Record
Medical Standard
Medical Times
Medico-Chirurgical Transactions
Methods of Molecular Medicine
Military Medicine
Monthly Bulletin of the Department of Health of the City of New York
Monthly Report of the Hospital and Health Board, Kansas City, Missouri
Mount Sinai Hospital Reports
New York Medical Journal
Northwest Medicine
Pennsylvania Medical Journal
Primary Care Update for OB/GYNS
Proceedings of Baylor University Medical Center
Public Health Reports
Review of Infectious Diseases
School
Science
Shield of Phil Kappa Psi
SMU Magazine
Texas State Journal of Medicine
Transactions of the American Clinical and Climatological Association
Transactions of the Epidemiological Society of London, New Series
Verhandl Kong Innere Medizinisch Wiesbaden
Vienna Klinische Wochenschrift

Journal Articles
- "Advertisements: Why Fear Rabies?" *Journal of the Missouri State Medical Association* 9, no. 12 (June 1913): vii.

- Albrecht, Heinrich, and Anton Ghon. "About the Etiology and Pathological Anatomy of Meningitis Cerebrospinalis Epidemica." *Vienna Klinische Wochenschrift* 14 (1901): 984–96.
- "Announcement: The Sophian-Hall-Alexander Laboratory." *Medical Herald* 31, no. 12 (December 1912): 673.
- Beebe, Alfred. "Diphtheria and Allied Pseudo-Membranous Inflammations, a Clinical and Bacteriological Study." *Medical Record* 42 (July 30 and August 6, 1892): 113–25, 141–47.
- Biggs, Hermann M. "The Development of the Research Laboratories." *Monthly Bulletin of the Department of Health of the City of New York* 1, no. 3 (March 1911): 54–56.
- Billings, J. S., Jr. "Cerebrospinal Meningitis in New York City during 1904 and 1905." *Journal of the American Medical Association* 46, no. 22 (June 2, 1906): 1670–76.
- "Biological Products: Establishments Licensed for the Propagation and Sale of Viruses, Serums, Toxins, and Analogous Products." *Public Health Reports* 28, no. 28 (July 11, 1913): 1445–47.
- Black, James Harvey. "Prophylactic Vaccination against Epidemic Meningitis." *Journal of the American Medical Association* 60, no. 17 (April 26, 1913): 1289–90.
- Black, James Harvey. "Prophylactic Vaccination against Epidemic Meningitis, a Supplementary Note." *Journal of the American Medical Association* 68, no. 24 (December 12, 1914): 2126.
- Bolduan, Charles F. "Cerebrospinal Meningitis from the Standpoint of Public Health." *Medical Times* 36, no. 7 (July 1908): 193–95.
- Bolduan, Charles F. "Over a Century of Health Administration in New York City." *Department of Health of the City of New York Monograph Series* 13 (March 1916): 23–24.

- "Book Reviews." *Cleveland Medical Journal* 12, no. 8 (August 1913): 573.
- "Book Reviews." *Northwest Medicine* 5, no. 8 (August 1913): 237.
- Bulloch, W. "Waldemar Mordecai Wolff Haffkine." *Journal of Pathology and Bacteriology* 34, no. 2 (1931): 125–29.
- "Bureau of Public Health and Marine Hospital Service." *Texas State Journal of Medicine* 7, no. 1 (May 1911): 31–32.
- Cartwright, K. "Microbiology and Laboratory Diagnosis." *Methods of Molecular Medicine* 67 (2001): 1–8.
- "Cerebrospinal Meningitis in Texas." *Public Health Reports* 27 no. 4 (January 26, 1912): 128.
- "Cerebro-spinal Meningitis in the United States, Etc." *Public Health Reports* 20, no. 15 (April 14, 1905): 655.
- "Cerebrospinal Meningitis: Cases and Deaths Reported by City Health Authorities for the Week Ended April 13, 1912." *Public Health Reports* 27, no. 17 (April 26, 1912): 651.
- "Cerebrospinal Meningitis: Cases and Deaths Reported by City Health Authorities for the Week Ended April 6, 1912." *Public Health Reports* 27, no. 18 (May 3, 1912): 619.
- "Communication: Serum Sickness." *Texas State Journal of Medicine* 7, no. 12 (April 1912): 335–36.
- Conner, Lewis A. "The Technique of Lumbar Puncture." *New York Medical Journal* 71 (May 12, 1900): 723–25.
- Cooper, E. A. "On the Relations of Phenol and Meta-Cresol to Proteins; Contribution to Our Knowledge of the Mechanism of Disinfection." *Biochemistry Journal* 6, no. 4 (1912): 362–87.
- Councell, Clara E. "War and Infectious Disease." *Public Health Reports* 56, no. 12 (March 21, 1941): 547–73.
- Coureuil, Mathieu, Olivier Join-Lambert, Hervé Lécuyer, Sandrine Bourdoulous, Stefano Marullo, and Xavier Nassif. "Pathogenesis of Meningococcemia." *Cold Spring Harbor Perspectives in Medicine* 3, no. 6 (June 2013): a012393.

- Danielson, Lothario, and Elias Mann. "The First American Account of Cerebrospinal Meningitis." *Review of Infectious Diseases* 5, no. 5 (September–October 1983): 969–72.
- Danielson, Lothario, and Elias Mann. "The History of a Singular and Very Mortal Disease Which Lately Made Its Appearance in Medfield." *Medical and Agricultural Register* 1 (1806): 65–69.
- Davis, David J. "Studies in Meningococcus Infections." *Journal of Infectious Diseases* 4, no. 4 (November 15, 1907): 558–681.
- Dowling, Harry Filmore. "Field, Ward, and Laboratory: Where the Infectious Disease Physician Worked." *Journal of Infectious Diseases* 153, no. 3 (March 1986): 390–96.
- "Dr. Ernest Franklin Robinson, Kansas Alpha, 1888." *Shield of Phi Kappa Psi* (November 1944): 160.
- "Dr. Hyde and Mr. Swope." KC History. Missouri Valley Special Collections. Kansas City Public Library. Accessed August 3, 2018. http://www.kchistory.org/week-kansas-city-history/dr-hyde-and-mr-swope.
- DuBois, Phebe L. "Differential Diagnosis and Treatment of Epidemic Cerebrospinal Meningitis." *Journal of the American Medical Association* 60, no. 11 (March 15, 1913): 820–22.
- "Epidemic Cerebrospinal Meningitis." *American Journal of Public Health* 3, no. 12 (December 1913): 1364.
- "Epidemic Meningitis: Editorial." *Medical Herald* 32, no. 2 (February 1913): 75–77.
- "Establishments Licensed for the Propagation and Sale of Viruses, Serums, Toxins, and Analogous Products." *Public Health Reports* 27, no. 2 (January 12, 1912): 40–41.
- "Frank C. Neff, MD, 1872–1947." *American Journal of Diseases of Children* 75, no. 4 (1948): 608–9.
- Flexner, Simon. "Accidents Following the Subdural Injection of the Antimeningitis Serum." *Journal of the American Medical Association* 60, no. 25 (June 21, 1913): 1937–40.

- Flexner, Simon. "Experimental Cerebrospinal Meningitis and Its Serum Treatment." *Journal of the American Medical Association* 47, no. 8 (August 25, 1906): 560–66.
- Flexner, Simon. "Experimental Cerebro-Spinal Meningitis in Monkeys." *Journal of Experimental Medicine* 9, no. 2 (March 14, 1907): 142–67.
- Flexner, Simon, and James Wesley Jobling. "Serum Treatment of Epidemic Cerebro-Spinal Meningitis." *Journal of Experimental Medicine* 10, no. 1 (January 1, 1908): 194–95.
- Freedman, Ben. "The First State Board of Health Laboratories in the United States." *Public Health Reports* 69, no. 9 (September 1954): 867–75.
- Frost, Wade Hampton. "Anti-meningitis Vaccination." *Public Health Reports* 28, no. 6 (February 7, 1913): 252–54.
- Frost, Wade Hampton. "Epidemic Cerebrospinal Meningitis: A Review of Its Etiology, Transmission, and Specific Therapy, with Reference to Public Measures for Its Control." *Public Health Reports* 27, no. 4 (January 26, 1912): 97–121.
- Gortler, Leon. "Merck in America: The First 70 Years from Fine Chemicals to Pharmaceutical Giant." *Bulletin of the History for Chemistry* 25, no.1 (2000): 1–9.
- Grady, Frank J. "Some Early American Reports on Meningitis." *Journal of the History of Medicine and Allied Sciences* 20, no. 1 (January 1, 1965): 27–32.
- Hall, Frank J. "Correspondence: Laboratory of Clinical Pathology." *Medical Herald* 32, no. 11 (November 1913): 431.
- Hand, Alfred, Jr. "A Critical Summary of the Literature on the Diagnostic and Therapeutic Value of Lumbar Puncture." *American Journal of the Medical Sciences* 120 (October 1900): 463–69.
- Hawgood, Barbara J. "Waldemar Mordecai Haffkine, CIE (1860–1930): Prophylactic Vaccination against Cholera

and Bubonic Plague in British India." *Journal of Medical Biography* 15, no. 1 (2007): 9–19.

- Heiman, Henry. "The Technics of Lumbar Puncture in Children: With Particular Reference to the Pressure of the Cerebrospinal Fluid." *Mount Sinai Hospital Reports* 5 (1905–1906): 114–23.
- "Henry Kendall Mulford." *Pennsylvania Medical Journal* 41, no. 2 (November 1937): 174.
- "History of the Kansas City General Hospital." *Jackson County Medical Journal* 26 (October 1, 1932): 11–25.
- Hospital and Health Board. "Contagious and Infectious Diseases Reported; Number and Deaths." *Monthly Report of the Hospital and Health Board, Kansas City, Missouri* 6, no. 1 (January 1912).
- Hospital and Health Board. "Contagious and Infectious Diseases Reported." *Monthly Report Hospital and Health Board, Kansas City, Missouri* 6, no. 3 (March 1912).
- Hospital and Health Board. "Contagious and Infectious Diseases Reported." *Monthly Report of the Hospital and Health Board, Kansas City, Missouri* 6, no. 4 (April 1912).
- Hospital and Health Board. "Contagious and Infectious Disease Reported." *Monthly Report of the Hospital and Health Board, Kansas City, Missouri* 6, no. 5 (May 1912).
- Hospital and Health Board. "Contagious Diseases Reported for the Year, 1912–1913." *Fifth Annual Report of the Hospital and Health Board of Kansas City, Missouri, for Fiscal Year April 16, 1912, to April 21, 1913.* Kansas City, MO: Hospital and Health Board, 1913, 87.
- Hospital and Health Board. "Medical Diseases—General Hospital, from April 16, 1912, to April 21, 1913." *Fifth Annual Report of the Hospital and Health Board of Kansas City, Missouri, for Fiscal Year April 16, 1912, to April 21, 1913, Inclusive.* Kansas City, MO: Hospital and Health Board, 1913, 135.
- "House Fly Catechism." *Bulletin of the Kansas State Board of Health* 7, no. 4 (April 1911): 75–76, 80.

- "In Memoriam, James Harvey Black, 1884–1958." *American Journal of Clinical Pathology* 32, no. 2 (August 1959): 172–73.

- "Interesting Announcement Is Made in This Issue by the H. K. Mulford Company Concerning Meningo-Bacterin (Meningococcus Vaccine)." *Medical Herald* 31, no. 4 (April 1912): 205.

- Jacoby, George W. "Lumbar Puncture of the Subarachnoid Space." *New York Medical Journal* 62 (December 28, 1895): 813–18.

- Jochmann, Georg. "Versuche zur Serodiagnostik und Serotherapie der epidemischen Genickstarre." *Deutsche Medizinische Wochenschrift* 1, no. 1 (1906): 788–93.

- "Kansas City General Hospital." Historic American Building Survey. National Park Service. HABS NO. MO-251. Accessed August 3, 2018. https://cdn.loc.gov/master/pnp/habshaer/mo/mo0500/mo0513/data/mo0513data.pdf.

- "Kansas City General Hospital." *Medical Herald* 31, no. 9 (September 1912): 472.

- Kere, J. W. "Organization of the Federal Public Health Service." *Public Health Reports* 28, no. 3 (January 17, 1913): 117–19.

- Kolle, Wilhelm, and August Wasserman. "Versuch zur Gewinnung und Wertbestimmung eines Meningococcenserums." *Deutsch Medizinische Wochenschrift* 32 (1906): 609–12.

- Kopetzky, Samuel Joseph. "Lumbar Puncture: A General Review of Its Value and Applicability." *American Journal of the Medical Sciences* 131 (April 1906): 648–74.

- Kramer, Simon Pendleton. "A Possible Source of Danger in the Use of Antimeningitis Serum." *Journal of the American Medical Association*, 60, no. 18 (May 3, 1913): 1348–51.

- Kramer, Simon Pendleton, and Rubert Boyce. "The Nature of Vaccine Immunity." *British Medical Journal* 2, no. 1714 (November 4, 1893): 989–90.

- Leck, Harriet. "The Helen Newberry Nurses' Home." *Modern Hospital* 10 (January to June 1918): 264–66.
- Long, J. H. "On the Work of the Council on Pharmacy and Chemistry of the American Medical Association." *Science* 32, no. 834 (December 23, 1910): 889–901.
- Low, Bruce R. "Epidemic Cerebrospinal Meningitis." *Transactions of the Epidemiological Society of London, New Series* 18 (January 20, 1899): 53–85.
- Madani, Kaivon. "Dr. Hans Christian Joachim Gram: Inventor of the Gram Stain." *Primary Care Update for OB/GYNS* 10, no. 5 (September–October 2003): 235–37.
- Marcet, Alexander. "History of a Singular Nervous or Paralytic Affection, Attended with Anomalous Morbid Sensations, Communicated by Dr. Marcet, Read Dec. 18, 1810." *Medico-Chirurgical Transactions* 2 (1811), 215–33.
- McIntosh, R. A. "Equine Encephalomyelitis from a Clinician's Point of View." *Canadian Journal of Comparative Medicine* 2, no. 8 (August 1938): 223–27.
- "Medical News." *Medical Herald* 32, no. 4 (April 1913): 163.
- "Medical News." *Medical Herald* 32, no. 11 (November 1913): 431.
- "Medical News, Alabama." *Journal of the American Medical Association* 68, no. 26 (June 29, 1912): 2037.
- "Medical News: Missouri: Serum Farm and Laboratory for Kansas City." *Journal of the American Medical Association* 59, no. 7 (August 17, 1912): 553.
- "Medical News, Texas." *Journal of the American Medical Association* 57, no. 11 (September 9, 1911): 909.
- "Minutes of the Meetings of the State Board of Health, January 24, 1913." State Board of Health of Missouri. *Thirty-First Annual Report of the State Board of Health and Bureau of Vital Statistics of Missouri 1913* (Jefferson City, MO: Hugh Stephens Printing Company, 1913): 12–14.
- "Missouri." *Journal of the American Institute of Homoeopathy* [sic] 1, no. 9 (September 1909): 444.

- "Missouri Biologic Laboratory." *Journal of the Missouri State Medical Association* 9, no. 10 (April 1913): 345.
- Mulford, H. K. "The Preparation of Diphtheria Antitoxic Serum." *Proceedings of the American Pharmaceutical Association at the Forty-Fourth Annual Meeting Held at Montreal, Canada, August 1896* (Baltimore, MD: American Pharmaceutical Association, 1896): 227–31.
- Müllener, Eduard-Rudolf. "Six Geneva Physicians on Meningitis." *Journal of the History of Medicine and Allied Sciences* 20, no. 1 (January 1965): 1–26.
- "M. Valleix." *Boston Medical and Surgical Journal* 52 (November 22, 1855): 352–53.
- Nash, Albert W. "'Epidemic Cerebrospinal Meningitis,' Official Transactions, Medical Association of the Southwest, Seventh Annual Session at Hot Springs, Ark., October 8–10, 1912." *Medical Herald* 32, no. 1 (January 1913): 8–11.
- Neal, Josephine B., and Harry L. Abramson. "A Comparison of Tricresol and Chloroform as a Preservative in Antimeningitis Serum." *Journal of the American Medical Association* 68, no. 14 (April 7, 1917): 1935–1937.
- "New and Nonofficial Remedies." *Journal of the American Medical Association* 60, no. 14 (April 5, 1913): 1074.
- "New Appointments." *Graduate Magazine of the University of Kansas* 14, no. 1 (October 1915): 22.
- "Normal College Graduates." *School* 11, no. 2 (September 19, 1899): 341.
- "Obituary, Dr. Meredith Clymer." *British Medical Journal* 1, no. 2159 (May 17, 1902): 1243.
- "Obituary [Dr. Rudolph Hermann Von Ezdorf]." *British Medical Journal* 2, no. 2917 (November 25, 1916): 746.
- "Obituaries [Dr. Rudolph Hermann Von Ezdorf]." *Military Medicine* 39 (1916): 453.
- Parascandola, John. "The Public Health Service and the Control of Biologics." *Public Health Reports* 110, no. 6 (November–December 1995): 774–75.

- Park, William Hallock. "The New Activities of the Research Laboratory of the Department of Health of the City of New York." *Monthly Bulletin of the Department of Health of New York City* 1–2 (1911–1912): 56–65.
- Parmelee, Arthur Hawley. "Epidemic Cerebrospinal Meningitis." *Journal of the American Medical Association* 60, no. 9 (March 1, 1913): 659–61.
- Pipkin, George R. "Report of Contagious Diseases." *Fourth Annual Report of the Hospital and Health Board of Kansas City, Missouri, for Fiscal Year April 17, 1911, to April 15, 1912, Inclusive* (Kansas City, MO: Hospital and Health Board, 1912), 148.
- Pope, Georgina F. "Bellevue Hospital, Past and Present." *American Journal of Nursing* 5, no. 1 (October 1904): 28–33.
- Pope, Georgina R. "Bellevue Hospital, Past and Present (Concluded)." *American Journal of Nursing* 5, no. 5 (February 1905): 291–96.
- Punton, John. "Hospitals of Kansas City," in D. M. Bone, *Kansas City Annual, 1907* (Kansas City, MO: Bishop Press, 1906): 61–64.
- Quincke, Heinrich. "Die Lumbalpunktion des Hydrocephalus." *Verhandl Kong Innere Medizinisch Wiesbaden* 10 (1891): 321–31.
- Quincke, Heinrich. "Über Lumbalpunktion." *Berliner Klinische Wochesnschrift* 32 (1895): 861–62, 929–33.
- Rackemann, Frances M. "Dr. Thomas Darlington." *Transactions of the American Clinical and Climatological Association* 58 (1946): lvii–lix.
- Raugewitz, Richard F. "The Horse Disease in Kansas, 1912–1913." *Emporia State Research Studies* 20, no. 2 (December 1917): 1–20.
- "Reliable Medicines." *Journal of the Missouri State Medical Association* 10, no. 5 (November 1913): 187.

- "Rev. Alexander Lewis, DD, '87." *Alumni Magazine, Carleton College, Northfield, Minnesota* 3, no.1 (May 1912): 17–21.
- Rice, George J., G. Weldon Tilley, and Peter A. Dysert. "A History of Pathology and Laboratory Medicine at Baylor University Medical Center." *Proceedings of Baylor University Medical Center* 17, no. 1 (January 2004): 42–55.
- Rodgers, Samuel U. "Kansas City General Hospital No. 2, a Historical Summary." *Journal of the National Medical Association* 54, no. 5 (September 1962): 525–639.
- Rothman, Philip. "Arthur Hawley Parmelee, MD, 1883–1961, Pioneer Pediatrician to the Newborn." *American Journal of the Diseases of Children* 103, no. 2 (1962): 197–200.
- "Rush Medical College." *Medical Standard* 22 (1899): 631.
- "Serum Farm in Kansas City." *Medical Herald* 31, no. 9 (September 1912): 471.
- Shutt, Edwin D. "The Saga of the Armour Family in Kansas City, 1870–1900." *Heritage of the Great Plains* 23 (Fall 1900).
- "Society Scintillations: Wichita, Sedgwick County Medical Society." *Medical Herald* 32, no. 2 (February 1913): 85.
- Sophian, Abraham. "Normal Serum Therapy." *Medical Herald* 31, no. 12 (December 1912): 615–20.
- Sophian, Abraham, and James Harvey Black. "Prophylactic Vaccination against Epidemic Meningitis." *Transactions of the Section on Pathology and Physiology of the American Medical Association at the Sixty-Third Annual Session, Held at Atlantic City, NJ, June 4 to 7, 1912* (1912): 59.
- Steers, William D. "Turner, Benjamin Weems." *Handbook of Texas Online.* Accessed February 9, 2018. https://tshaonline.org/handbook/online/articles/ftu15.
- Thayer, Alfred Edward. "The Dallas Epidemic of Meningitis; Preliminary Note on the Laboratory Work." *Texas State Journal of Medicine* 7, no. 11 (March 1912): 305–7.

- "The Function of Research in Municipal Health Administration." *Monthly Bulletin of the Department of Health of the City of New York* 1, no. 3 (March 1911): 51–53.

- "The General Hospital a School for Nurses, Colored Department," in *Crisis, A Record of the Darker Races* 9, no. 2 (December 1914): 56.

- "The New Charter." *Kansas City Medical Index-Lancet* 31, no. 346 (October 1908): 370–71.

- "The Sophian-Hall-Alexander Laboratories." *Journal of the Oklahoma State Medical Association* 5, no. 3 (January 1913): 391.

- "Transfer of Agency." New and Nonofficial Remedies. *Journal of the American Medical Association* 61, no. 15 (October, 11, 1913): 1377.

- Vieusseux, Gaspard. "Mémoire sur la maladie qui a règne à Genève, au printemps de 1805." *Journal de Médecine, Chirurgie, Pharmacie, Etc.*, tome xii (1806): 163–82.

- Von Ezdorf, Rudolph H. "Cerebrospinal Meningitis in Texas." *Public Health Reports* 27, no. 8 (February 23, 1912): 271–72.

- Wall, Cecil. "On Acute Cerebro-Spinal Meningitis Caused by the Diplococcus Intracellularis of Weichselbaum: A Clinical Study." *Medico-Chirurgical Transactions* 86 (1903): 77–79.

- Wassermann, August. "Über die Bisherigen Erfahrungen mit dem Meningococcen-Heilserum bei Genickstarre-kranken." *Deutsch Medizinische Wochenschrift* 33 (1907): 1585–87.

- Watson, David, Daniel M. Muser, James W. Jacobson, and J. Verhoef. "A Brief History of the Pneumococcus in Biomedical Research: A Panoply of Scientific Discovery." *Clinical Infectious Diseases* 17, no. 5 (November 1993): 913–24.

ABOUT THE AUTHORS

MARGARET R. O'LEARY, MD

D r. Margaret Rose O'Leary was born in Indianapolis, Marion County, Indiana, in 1952 as the second eldest of the five children of Dr. Gerald Philip Wiedman (1924–1995), an internist and cardiologist, and Margaret "Peg" Rose McGrath (1926–2008). Dr. O'Leary graduated from the Anna Head School (now the Head-Royce School, Oakland, Alameda County, California) in 1970; earned a bachelor's degree in religion from Smith College (Northampton, Hampshire County, Massachusetts) in 1974 and a bachelor's degree in zoology from the University of California, Berkeley (Berkeley, Alameda County, California) in 1976; and received her medical degree from the George Washington University School of Medicine (Washington, DC) in 1980. She completed her emergency medicine residency at the Georgetown University Medical Center, George Washington University Medical Center, and Maryland Institute of Emergency Medical Services program (1980–1984) and became one of the earliest residency-trained and board-certified emergency physicians in the United States. She served as an assistant professor of emergency medicine and emergency department attending physician at both the George Washington University Medical Center (1984–1986) and the University of Chicago Hospitals (1987–1988) and as an attending emergency physician at Saint

Therese Medical Center in Waukegan, Lake County, Illinois (1988–1989). She thereafter became a senior consulting writer at the Joint Commission on Accreditation of Healthcare Organizations (now the Joint Commission) in Oakbrook Terrace, DuPage County, Illinois (1988–1995), where she authored the *Primer on Indicator Development and Application*; *The Measurement Mandate*; *Clinical Performance Data*; and *Lexikon: Dictionary of Health Care Terms, Organizations, and Acronyms*. In 1995, she returned to clinical emergency medicine as an attending physician at Northwest Community Hospital in Arlington Heights, Cook County, Illinois (1995–1998). In 1999, she earned her master of business administration degree at Benedictine University in Lisle, DuPage County, Illinois, and on graduation, she joined its academic faculty as an associate professor of management and the director of its MBA programs (1999–2002). After the attack on the United States on September 11, 2001, she accepted a large, unsolicited grant from the Grace Bersted Foundation, which she applied to the establishment of the Suburban Emergency Management Project (SEMP) in DuPage County, Illinois (2001–2010). The SEMP conducted community-based emergency preparedness activities for two years and produced three books (*The First 72 Hours*, *The Dictionary of Homeland Security*, and *Measuring Disaster Preparedness*), eight years of the popular monthly *Securitas Magazine* and the weekly *SEMP Biots*. Dr. O'Leary served on the boards of the American Academy of Emergency Medicine (Milwaukee, Milwaukee County, Wisconsin) and the Girl Scouts of DuPage County (Naperville, DuPage County, Illinois). Around 2008, Dr. O'Leary moved with her husband to the Kansas City area, where she enjoys gardening, playing her cellos, and writing.

DENNIS S. O'LEARY, MD

Dr. Dennis Sophian O'Leary was born in Kansas City, Jackson County, Missouri, in 1938 as the eldest of the two sons of Theodore Morgan O'Leary (1910–2001), a writer, editor, sports correspondent, and literary critic, and Emily Sophian (1913–1994), the daughter of Dr. Abraham Sophian, an individual in this book. Dr. O'Leary graduated from Shawnee Mission High School (Shawnee Mission, Johnson County, Kansas) in 1956; earned his bachelor's degree with a major in social relations from Harvard College in 1960; and received his medical degree from Cornell University Medical College in Manhattan in 1964. He then completed internal medicine residencies at the University of Minnesota Medical Center (1964–1966) and the University of Rochester Medical Center (1966–1968). Thereafter, he served in the United States Army Medical Corps as the director of the blood-coagulation laboratory at the Walter Reed Army Institute of Research (1968–1971) in Washington, DC, attaining the rank of major. He then joined the internal medicine faculty of the George Washington University Medical Center in Washington, DC, in 1971, rising in rank from assistant professor to full professor in 1979. In 1974, he was appointed acting medical director of the George Washington University Hospital, a position he held until 1986. He was appointed dean for clinical affairs at the George Washington University Hospital in 1978, a position he also held until 1986. In 1981, he achieved fame as the spokesman for the George Washington University Hospital following the attempted assassination of US president Ronald Reagan, reporting to the news media daily on the president's and Press Secretary James Brady's recovery from their wounds in the George Washington University Hospital. He subsequently served as the president of the Medical Society of the District of Columbia (1983). In 1986, he became president of the Joint Commission on Accreditation of Healthcare Organizations (now The Joint Commission) in Chicago, a position he held for twenty-one years, at which time he retired as president emeritus of the organization. In 1992, he was elected to the Institute of Medicine (now the National Academy of Medicine). He has served on many boards, including the National Advisory Council of the Agency for Healthcare Research and Quality (2001–2005), the Defense Health Board of the US Department of Defense (2009–2013), the National Patient Safety Foundation and the Lucian Leape Institute (2008–2013), the Truman Medical Center Board of Directors in Kansas City, Missouri (2008–2013), and the Institute for Healthcare Improvement (2008–2012). Around 2008, Dr. O'Leary moved with his wife to his childhood home near Kansas City to run his family's farms and estate. He closely follows all sports, reads novels, and devours crossword puzzles.

INDEX

bold denotes photo

A

Aaron, Gertrude Claire, 90n8
Adamson, Effie Lucinda Sloan,
     112, 113, 124n37
African Americans
     Old Hospital as turned over to,
          190–191n17
     who contracted cerebrospinal
          meningitis in Kansas City,
          40, 113–114, 115, 131, 152
Albrecht, Heinrich, 6, 22n23
Alexander, Elliot Richie, 165,
     167, 169, 175, 180, 186, 188–
     189n4, 209
Alexander, James Ritchie,
     188–189n4
Alexander, Sarah Amanda
     Vanderhoef, 188–189n4
American Biologic Company, 58,
     147, 166, 181, 208
*American Journal of Public
     Health*, 186
American Medical Association,
     Council on Pharmacy
     and Chemistry, 181–182,
     197–198n62
     antimeningitis serum

administration of, 111,
     132, **185**
advice to obtain supply of, 51
clinical tests for, 112–113
development of, 11
discontinuation of Flexner's
     free distribution of, 46
establishments licensed to sell,
     97n36
Flexner's free distribution of,
     13, 44, 45
increased demand for, 132–133
intraspinal injection of, 12,
     13, 177
manufacture of, 47, 48, 84,
     97n37, 166
praise for, 46
shortage of, 133, 134
St. Louis City Hospital
     physicians' first use of,
     64–65n44
subcutaneous injection of,
     11–12, 73, 82, 105, 174
use of tricresol in, 177–178
Armour, Charles Watson, 35, 53n5
assistant surgeons, 85, 97–98n38,
     98n41
Aves, Charles S., 71–72n69

249

Aves, Frederick Worley (Fred W.),
50, 71–72n69
Aves, Jessie Olivia Hughes,
71–72n69

B

Barbeau, William Joseph
("Jap"), 45
Barbeau, William Joseph, Jr., 45
Barnes, Alfred E., Jr., 211n5
Barnes, Alfred Edward, 211n5
Barnes, Asa Beebe Cross, 211n5
Barnes, Catherine (Kate) Beebe
Cross, 202–205, 211n5
Barton, W. H., 115
Baylor University College of
Medicine, 103, 118n3,
161–162n30
Beardsley, Henry Mahan,
99–100n50
Beggs, Rachel, 114
Bellevue Hospital, 9, 22n25
Bierer, Octavia H., 191–192n19
Biewend, Mathilde Julie Henriette,
20n17
Biggs, Hermann Michael, 9,
25n32, 26–27n35, 27–28n37,
30–31n48
Biggs, Joseph Hunt, 26–27n35
Biggs, Melissa A., 26–27n35
Black, James Adam, 161–162n30
Black, James Harvey, 149, 161–
162n30, 162n34, 162n35,
167, 176
Black, Mary Nancy Murphy,
161–162n30
Board of Hospital and Health of
Kansas City, Missouri, 35
Bolduan, Charles Frederick, 9–10,
29n39

Bolduan, Julianne Caroline
Dreibholz, 29n39
Bolduan, William, 29n39
Boppert, Louis Martin, 87–88,
100n55
Boppert, Louis, Sr., 100n55
Boppert, Margaret E. Wagner,
100n55
Briggs, Imogene O., 56–57n14
Britt, Leila, 69n61
Broom, Mary, 131–132
Brown, Cordelia, 74n74
Brown, Ruth Frances, 70–71n67
bubonic plague vaccine, 95n23
Buchanan-Andrews County
Medical Society, 174
Bunte, Elise Mellies, 69n62
Bunte, Herman E., 69n62
Bunte, Louis Edward, 49,
69n62, 175
Burke, Foster Wand, Sr., 175,
194n39
Burke, John Lewis, 194n39
Burke, Mary Frances Moss,
194n39
Burton, W. H., 130
Busher, George, 114

C

Cabot, Richard, 76n78
Cain, Helen, 130
Campbell, William, 114
Carnes, Margaret, 72–73n71
Carpenter, Sallie Willis, 53n6
Carroll, James, 85
case count, 10, 12, 134, 149
case fatality rates, 12
Castelaw, David Marion,
191–192n19
Castelaw, Josephine English,
191–192n19

251

Engel, Josef, 21n19
Engelsdorff, Herma, 29n39
Ennis, John William, 136n5
Ennis, Leonora Ann, 136n5
Ennis, Marie, 130, 136n5
"Epidemic Cerebrospinal
   Meningitis: A Review of
   Its Etiology, Transmission,
   and Specific Therapy, with
   Reference to Pubic Measures
   for Its Control" (Frost), 85
"Epidemic Cerebrospinal
   Meningitis" (Nash), 173–174
"Epidemic Cerebrospinal
   Meningitis" (Parmelee), 177
Epidemic Cerebrospinal Meningitis
   (Sophian), 180, 184–186
Ewald, Katherine F., 23n26
Eyman, Alice Thurza Prickett,
   73–74n73
Eyman, Elmer Vail, 50, 73–74n73
Eyman, Franklin Pierce, 73–74n73

F

Farbwerke Vormals Meister, Lucius
   und Bruning, 97n36
Farrell, Eddie, 131
Fayles, General, 131
Federal Public Health Service
   (US Treasury Department),
   97–98n38
Felix, Arthur A., 155–156n8
Felix, Emilie Leitner, 155–156n8
Felix, Estelle, 67n53, 155–156n8
Felix, Eugenia, 155–156n8
Felix, Eugenie (Jane), 155–156n8
Felix, Eva, 155–156n8
Felix, Flora, 155–156n8
Felix, Joseph, 155–156n8
Felix, Louis, 155–156n8
Felix, Pauline, 155–156n8

Felix, Sarah, 155–156n8
Ferro, Francisco, 114
*Fifth Annual Report of the
   Hospital and Health Board of
   Kansas City for Fiscal Year
   April 16, 1912 to April 21,
   193*, 182, **182**, 183
Finn, Thomas Martin, 216n27
Fisher, Albert, 130, 132
Flexner, Esther Abraham,
   25–26n33
Flexner, Moritz (Morris),
   25–26n33
Flexner, Simon, 9, 11, 12–13, 25–
   26n33, 25n32, 64–65n44, 81,
   112, 178, 193n34
fly, common house, 212n8
Foote, Grace Humphrey, 213n11
Fort Worth, Texas, deaths from
   cerebrospinal meningitis, 112
Fortschritte der Medizin
   (Weichselbaum), 6
Foster, Frances Boyd, 24–25n30
Fraatz, Emilie Adolfine Sophie,
   20n17
Frank, Robert Tilden, 215n20
Freiberg, Edwig Emma Franziska,
   20n17
Freud, Sigmund, 101–102n59
Friedländer, Carl, 21–22n20
Frost, Henry Rutledge, Jr., 98n40
Frost, Sabra Jane Walker, 98n40
Frost, Wade Hampton, 85,
   98n40, 176
Fuller, Josephine, 132

G

Garesche (Gareschi), Virginia
   Margaret, 19–20n13
Gaynor, William Jay, 23–24n28
German Hospital, 102n62

meningococcus, 6, 7, 11, 80, 144–145, 162n34, 219

Mercer, Joseph Hooker, 189–190n8

Merck, George Friedrich, 212–213n10

Merck and Company, 212–213n10

Miller, Frances ("Frankie") A., 53–54n7

Mitchell, Louis, 107

Moffet, Alberta F., 102n62

Moody, Ruth Adaline, 57n16

Morris, Joel T., 137n13

Morris, Margaret J. Simpson, 137n13

Morris, William Clay, 132, 137n13

Morrison, Nettie A., 32–33n60

mortality rate
    compared to case fatality rate, 12
    statistics of, 5, 7, 7–8*t*, 9

Motley, John Glenn, 53n6

Motley, Louisa Perry, 53n6

Motley, William Perry, 35, 53n5, 53n6, 141, 143, 190–191n17, 220

Mulford, Adeline Brooks Nieukirk, 68n55

Mulford, Henry Kendall, 48, 68n55

Mulford, Joseph Lewis, 68n55

Murphy, Franklin E., 50, 74n74, 130

Murphy, Hugh C., 74n74

Murphy, Martha J. Cook, 74n74

Mycobacterium tuberculosis, 5, 21n18

N

Nash, Albert Ware, 81–82, 91–92n13, 103, 173–174

Nash, Mary Frances Hobbs, 91–92n13

Nash, Thomas Fletcher, 91–92n13

Neal, James Park, 38, 40, 41, 56–57n14

Neal, Joseph Marion, 56–57n14

Neal, March Virginia Humphrey, 56–57n14

Neelsen, Friedrich, 21n18

Neff, Andrew Jackson, 121n17

Neff, Ann Hassleton Chaffee, 121n17

Neff, Frank Chaffee, 107, 121n17

Neisseria meningitides, 6, 7, 13, 16n4

Nesbit, Edwin Lightner, 160n27, 208

Nesbit, Joseph C., 160n27

Nesbit, Rebecca M. Lightner, 160n27

New York City Board of Health, 9, 10, 27–28n37, 47, 84, 134

New York City, cerebrospinal meningitis epidemics in, 5, 7–9, 201–202

Nielson, Rose Emma, 91–92n13

Nixon, John, 136n9

Nixon, John Wesley, 131–132, 136n9

Nixon, Martha Ramsey, 136n9

normal serum therapy, 170–173

North, Elisha, 3, 16–17n5

North, Joseph, Jr., 16–17n5

North, Lucy Cole, 16–17n5

Northrup, William P., 25n32

Norton, Guy, 132

nose and throat cleansing, as prevention, 108

nurses, training school for, 38, 60n20

Nye, Charlotte Crosby Thomas, 100–101n57

Nye, Elisha, 100–101n57

R

Rau, Anna, 125n38
Rau, Gus, 125n38
Rau, Herbert Julius, 112, 125n38
Rau, Kurt Ernst, 112, 125n38
Red Cross Hospital, 102n62
Reed, J. A., 53–54n7
Reefer, Beatrice, 123–124n32
Research Laboratory (New York
    City Board of Health), 9, 11,
    27–28n37, 47, 48, 148, 178
Revised Statutes of the State of
    Missouri (1909), 41–42, 49
Rider, Mary ("Polly"), 17–18n8
RMS *Titanic*, 143
Robinson, Cornelia, 61–62n30
Robinson, David Hamilton,
    68–69n60
Robinson, Ernest Franklin, 49, 50,
    68–69n60
Robinson, Fred, 131
Robinson, George Wilse, 41, 42–
    43, 61–62n30
Robinson, George Woodson,
    61–62n30
Robinson, Henrietta Beach,
    68–69n60
Robinson, John Lincoln, 50,
    75n76, 130
Robinson, Levi, 75n76
Robinson, Mary F. Bradley, 75n76
Rockefeller, Eliza Davison, 26n34
Rockefeller, John Davison, Sr.,
    25–26n33, 26n34
Rockefeller, William Avery, 26n34
Rockefeller Institute for Medical
    Research, 9, 11, 25–26n33,
    26n34, 46, 47, 112
Rogers, Jennie Mason, 52–53n4
Rogers, Stuart Hayden, 73n72

Rokitansky, Carl Freiherr von,
    21n19
rooming houses. *See also* lodging
    houses
    cases of cerebrospinal
        meningitis from people in,
        108, 109
    described, 89n3
    fumigation and disinfecting of,
        85, 87
    sanitary measures and use of
        prophylaxis at, 127
    thorough cleaning of, 183,
        198n65
Rourke, Daniel Lawrence,
    59–60n19
Rush, Benjamin, 16–17n5

S

Salmonella enterica typhi, as cause
    of typhoid fever, 94–95n22
Sanders, St. Elmo, 99–100n50
Schorer, Bertha Wallschlaeger,
    193n34
Schorer, Edwin ("Teddy") Henry,
    170, 172, 193n34
Schorer, Robert Rudolph, 193n34
Schott, George, 71n68
Schott, Harry Johnson, 50, 71n68
Schott, Mary Cynthia (Mamie)
    Johnson, 71n68
Schulz, Alwiena August Zedler,
    194n38
Schulz, Frederick Bernhard,
    194n38
Schulz, Gustav Bernhard, 175,
    194n38
Semple, John McFarland,
    24–25n30
Sergeant, Josephine Alice,
    23–24n28

261

St. George's Hospital (Pest House), 54–55n9

St. Joseph (St. Joseph's) Hospital, 45, 65–66n45, 102n62

St. Luke's Hospital, 102n62

Stafford, Mary C., 133

Starr, Elizabeth Carrie, 117–118n1

State Board of Health (Missouri), 42, 49

Steele, Baylis, 216n27

Stone, Charles Prescott, 59n18

Stone, Ella Linette Aldrich, 59n18

Stone, Murry (Murray) Chaffee, 38, 59n18, 83

Stricker, Salomon, 117–118n1

Strohm, Margaret, 115

Stubbs, Walter Roscoe, 189–190n8

subarachnoid space, 32n56

subcutaneous injection
  of antimeningitis serum, 11–12, 73, 82, 105, 174
  of Meningo-Bacterin, 158n19

swabbers, 104, 118–119n5

Swinney, Edward Fletcher, 35

Swiss Serume and Vaccine Institute, 97n36

Swope, Frances Ann Hunton, 55–56n10

Swope, John Brevett, 55–56n10

Swope, Thomas Hunton, 37, 55–56n10, 57–58n17, 63n38

T

Taft, Eleanor Mabel, 59n18

Taylor, Harriet Rachael ("Isabella"), 156–157n10

Taylor, William E., 211n5

Teachenor, Frank Randall, 50, 72n70

Teachenor, Mary Catherine Givaudin, 72n70

Teachenor, Richard Bennington, 72n70

Texas State Journal of Medicine, 149

Thayer, Alfred Edward, 103, 104, 105, 117–118n1, 118–119n5, 119–120n10, 149

Thayer, Elizabeth Russell Cox, 117–118n1

Thayer, Stephen Howard, Sr., 117–118n1

thecal sac, 32n56

Traité de la Nouvelle Méthode d'Inoculer La Petite Vérole (Vieusseux), 15n2

transmissible, use of term, x

A Treatise on a Malignant Epidemic Commonly Called Spotted Fever (North), 16–17n5

tricresol, 177–178, 195–196n47

tubercular meningitis, cause of, 5

tuberculosis
  cases of in Kansas City March 1912, 138n27
  cause of, 5

Tuck, Elizabeth, 59n18

Turner, Annie Dorothy Krause, 72–73n71

Turner, Benjamin Weems, 50, 72–73n71

Turner, Francis Williamson, 72–73n71

typhoid fever, cause of, 94–95n22

typhoid vaccine, 94–95n22, 96n27

U

University Hospital, 102n62

University of Dallas Medical Department, 118n3

urotropin, 85, 99n45, 108, 144

US Treasury Department
   federal license for biologics,
      166, 186
   Federal Public Health Service,
      97–98n38

V

vaccination, 91n11, 144, 145–147,
   149, 162n34, 167, 174, 176,
   220. *See also* "Prophylactic
   Vaccination against Epidemic
   Meningitis" (Sophian and
   Black); *specific vaccines*
Valleix, François Louis Isidore, 4,
   18–19n11
Van Cott, Joshua, 25n32
VanAtta, John (?), 95--96n26
VanAtta, John Roberts, 83,
   95--96n26, 96n27, 145–146,
   157n16
VanAtta, Mary Eleanor,
   95--96n26
Vieusseux, Gaspard, 1–2, 15n2
violet-colored pinprick (petechial)
   rash, 16n4
vital-statistic reporting law, 41–
   42, 49

W

Waco, Texas, deaths from
   cerebrospinal meningitis in,
   79, 112
Walton, Walter, 110
Ware, Lillian Bell, 68n55
Wasserman, August von, 11
Watson, John, 110
Watson, John B., 131
Wehmeyer, John, 132
Weichselbaum, Anton, 6, 14,
   21n19, 22n23

Weicker, Anna Marie Elisabeth
   Momberger, 212–213n10
Weicker, Johann Adam Theodor
   (Theodore), 207, 212–213n10,
   213–214n12, 213n11
Weicker, Ludwig Christian,
   212–213n10
Weigert, Carl, 21–22n20
Weissenborn, Lena, 188–189n4
Welch, James A., 114, 115
Welch, William Henry, 25–26n33
Wheeler, Bertan Henry, 110,
   122n26
Wheeler, Henry T., 122n26
Wheeler, John Cummings, 53–54n7
Wheeler, Katharine ("Kate")
   Copenhaver, 53–54n7
Wheeler, Marie E. Langren,
   122n26
Wheeler, Walter Sewell, 35–36, **36**,
   38, 41, 53–54n7, 79, 81, 85, 87,
   97n37, 106, 107, 111, 127–129,
   132, 134, 144, 146, 147,
   148, 150–151, 156–157n10,
   169, 182, 183, 198n65, 201,
   202, 208
White, Frank, 115
Whitney, Mary Eleanor, 57–58n17
Wichita, Sedgwick County Medical
   Society, 174–175
Wiedenmann, John F., 216n27
Wilde, Harriet Miriam, 213n11
Williams, Anna, 27–28n37
Williams, Jack, 84, 87
Wilson, William E., 57–58n17
Wolfe, Katherine, 133
Wright, Almroth Edward, 83,
   94–95n22, 95n23
Wyandotte County Medical Society
   in Kansas, 144

Y

yellow fever, 117–118n1
Young, Hugh Hampton, 72–73n71

Z

Ziehl, Franz, 21n18
Ziehl-Neelsen stain, 21n18